The
Healthiest Diet
on the Planet

Previous National Bestselling McDougall Books:

The McDougall Plan

McDougall's Medicine: A Challenging Second Opinion

The McDougall Health Supporting Cookbook, Volume 1

The McDougall Health Supporting Cookbook, Volume 2

The McDougall Program: 12 Days to Dynamic Health

The McDougall Program for Maximum Weight Loss

The New McDougall Cookbook

The McDougall Program for Women

The McDougall Program for a Healthy Heart

The McDougall Quick and Easy Cookbook

Dr. McDougall's Digestive Tune-Up

The Starch Solution

Contact Information:

Dr. McDougall's Health and Medical Center
PO Box 14039, Santa Rosa, CA 95402
Telephone: (707) 538-8609   FAX: (707) 538-0712
Book orders: http://www.drmcdougall.com/books_tapes.html
E-mail: office@drmcdougall.com
On the web: http://www.drmcdougall.com
Residential program: (800) 941-7111 / (707) 538-8609

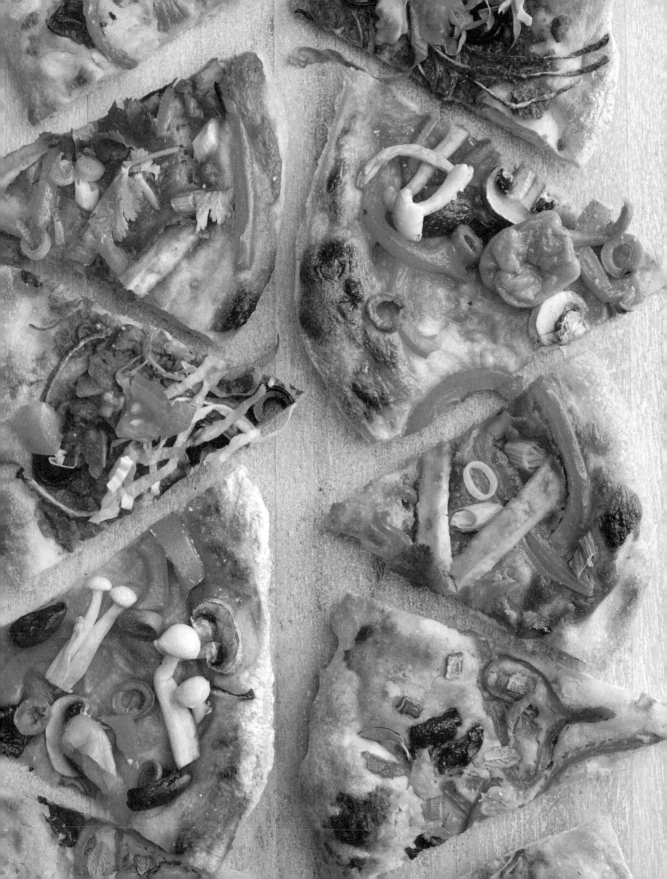

Why the Foods You Love—
Pizza, Pancakes, Potatoes,
Pasta, and More—
Are the Solution to Preventing
Disease and Looking and
Feeling Your Best

The
Healthiest Diet
on the Planet

John McDougall, M.D.
Recipes by Mary McDougall

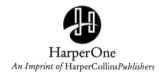

HarperOne
An Imprint of HarperCollinsPublishers

HarperOne

HarperCollins books may be purchased for educational, business, or sales promotional use. For information, please email the Special Markets Department at SPsales@harpercollins.com.

FIRST EDITION

Recipe photographs by Jennifer Davick Photography

Interior Design by Ralph Fowler

Red Light, Green Light: Dr. McDougall's Guide to What We Should and Shouldn't Eat layout by Colleen Teitgen Design and Ralph Fowler

Library of Congress Cataloging-in-Publication Data

Names: McDougall, John A.
Title: The healthiest diet on the planet : why the foods you love—pizza, pancakes, potatoes, pasta, and more—are the solution to preventing disease and looking and feeling your best / John McDougall.
Description: First editon. | New York, NY : HarperOne, [2016]
Identifiers: LCCN 2016028324 (print) | LCCN 2016031836 (ebook) | ISBN 9780062426765 (hardback) | ISBN 9780062426789 (e-book)
Subjects: LCSH: Nutrition. | Health—Nutritional aspects. | Diet. | BISAC: HEALTH & FITNESS / Nutrition. | COOKING / Health & Healing / General. | HEALTH & FITNESS / Diets.
Classification: LCC RA784 .M3952 2016 (print) | LCC RA784 (ebook) | DDC 613.2—dc23
LC record available at https://lccn.loc.gov/2016028324

ISBN 978–0–06–2426765

16 17 18 19 20   RRD   10 9 8 7 6 5 4 3 2 1

Contents

This book is dedicated to our grandchildren:

Jaysen Wilson
Ben Wilson
Ryan Wilson
Sam McDougall
Chloe McDougall
Nolan McDougall
Logan McDougall

And all other grandchildren

The world is ours to save. The Healthiest Diet on the Planet will change our present course of global warming, environmental destruction, and species extinction, hopefully overnight.

1

There Are Lies and Damned Lies

Damned lies harm the public and planet Earth. In June 2015, the *Journal of the American Medical Association,* in a reckless opinion piece, called for the U.S. Department of Agriculture (USDA) and the Department of Health and Human Services (DHHS) to remove an upper limit on the intake of total dietary fat in its most recent *Dietary Guidelines for Americans 2015–2020.*[1] To my dismay, the authors of this article also applauded the "elimination of dietary cholesterol as a 'nutrient of concern.'"

The facts behind the journal's article are deeply flawed and grossly and irresponsibly skewed in favor of the meat, poultry, dairy, fish, and egg industries, public enemies when it comes to our health. For most Americans, these animal-derived foods are the primary sources of cholesterol and fat. The next largest source of dietary fat is vegetable oil (such as canola, coconut, corn, flaxseed, olive, and safflower). Although the human body does require fat, especially during times of extreme food shortage, plants provide all of the essential fats we need. Removing an upper limit on fat intake promotes obesity, heart disease, type 2 diabetes, and common cancers (breast, colon, and prostate). Furthermore, regardless of its source, *the fat you eat is the fat you wear.* So-called good fat like olive oil is no more attractively worn around people's waistlines than bad fat from lard.

Lying about our dietary needs is inexcusable. Rather than encouraging the consumption of animal products and vegetable oils, as the authors of this opinion piece suggest, the USDA and the DHHS need to classify these foods as toxic, and the federal government needs to regulate the production, marketing, and selling of these foods in the same way it regulates tobacco and alcohol. Seven decades of personal and professional experience have taught me that these foods will kill you, slowly and surely.

The Problem: "Improvements" in Our Diet

During most of human existence, the average life expectancy was an astonishing twenty-five years or less. To date, no prehistoric remains have been found of people older than fifty years.[2] With few exceptions, war, accidents, starvation, or infection ended lives before any telltale signs of aging—graying of the hair, wrinkling of the skin, memory loss, a reduction of strength and loss of muscle mass, and decreased visual acuity—appeared. With the development of civilization, however, people learned to master their environment and to better protect themselves; with these advances some people survived to a ripe old age. Passages from the Bible, written more than twenty-five hundred years ago, report that death from old age typically occurred between seventy and eighty (Psalm 90:10), while other passages predict a maximum life-span of 120 years (Genesis 6:3).

In the nineteenth century, the introduction of immunizations, better nutrition, proper sanitation, and possibly antibiotics resulted in an unprecedented boost in life-span. Life expectancy has increased

The History of Average Life-Spans (in Years)[3]

Prehistoric Era	25
Classical Greece	28
Classical Rome	28
Medieval England	29
United States in 1800	37
United States in 1900	47
United States in 1950	68
United States in 2002	77
United States in 2016	79
Japan in 2002	82
All Adventists in 2002	85
Vegetarian Adventists	87

since the beginning of the twentieth century from age forty-seven to the current seventy-nine years by effectively stopping infectious diseases that killed people from birth to young adulthood.[4] At the same time, nutrient-deficiency diseases that were once considered life-threatening, like scurvy, beriberi, pellagra, and goiters, have been reduced through public nutritional advice focused on eating more fruits and vegetables (and secondarily on taking vitamin and mineral supplements).

By the middle of the twentieth century, it seemed we were well on our way to enjoying a lifetime of sustainable good health and remarkable longevity. But it didn't turn out that way. Not even close. Because chronic and degenerative diseases like obesity, heart disease, strokes, type 2 diabetes, arthritis, and cancers quickly replaced nutritional deficiencies and infectious diseases as the predominant causes of disability and death in the country.

How did this happen? What changed? How did we go from achieving the healthiest and longest life-span in the history of humankind to suddenly becoming chronically sick and in constant danger of dropping dead before reaching our golden years?

The answer is simple—startlingly, maddeningly simple. The food industries got involved.

The Food Industries and the *McGovern Report*

Jumping on the national health bandwagon, the food industries started pushing meat, poultry, fish, and eggs as invaluable sources of protein, and dairy foods as essential for our calcium needs, which, both the meat and dairy industries claimed, were cornerstones of a healthy diet, even though protein and calcium deficiencies were nonexistent problems (except during starvation, and then all nutrients are deficient).[5] The meat and dairy industries were so successful at hawking protein and calcium in the first half of the twentieth century that, by the 1960s, the average consumer was convinced—absolutely certain—that protein and calcium were the most vital of all nutrients for a healthy body and a long life, despite the absence of any scientific or nutritional research to support such a claim. In fact, the research at the time was beginning to link chronic and acute diseases with the excessive consumption of meat and dairy, specifically the outrageously high concentrations of saturated fat and cholesterol, and the absence of dietary fiber, essential vitamins and minerals, and other plant-derived nutrients. It is no accident that the death rate for coronary heart disease in the United States rose steadily during this period, reaching a peak in 1968 (238.5 people per 100,000 population).[6] It was not uncommon for Americans during the mid-twentieth century to die from heart attacks in their fifties and sixties.

At the same time, pockets of the country were suffering from hunger and malnutrition, most notably in the rural South, where emaciated children were testing positive for diseases that had only existed in underdeveloped countries. Recognizing this downturn in America's health, the U.S. Senate took formal action. Between 1968 and 1977, the Senate convened on numerous occasions its Select Committee on Nutrition and Human Needs, which ultimately produced the country's first *Dietary Goals for the United States,* then known as the *McGovern Report,* in recognition of George McGovern, the Democratic senator from South Dakota and chair of the committee.[7] These new guidelines on eating were expected to have health-changing effects similar to the *1964 Surgeon General's Report on Smoking and Health,* which helped reduce the prevalence of smoking cigarettes from 50 percent of the adult population in the 1970s to less than 20 percent today.[8]

Although it initially focused on hunger and malnutrition, the committee expanded its scope to include all aspects of nutrition, from eating too little to eating too much. In doing so, the committee took on obesity, heart disease, diabetes, high blood pressure, and certain kinds of cancer. "There is a great deal of evidence and it continues to accumulate, which strongly implicates and, in some instances, proves that the major causes of death and disability in the United States are related to the diet we eat," wrote Dr. D. Mark

Hegsted, of the Harvard School of Public Health, in the *McGovern Report*. "I include coronary artery disease, which accounts for nearly half the deaths in the United States, several of the most important forms of cancer, hypertension, diabetes and obesity as well as other chronic diseases."[9]

Through its findings, the committee urged the American public to cut back on fat, cholesterol, simple sugars, and refined and processed grains in favor of complex carbohydrates (which were once commonly known as starches), rich in dietary fiber. In lay terms, the committee told people to stop eating so much meat, poultry, eggs, and dairy products and to start eating more fruits, vegetables, and whole grains.

"The question to be asked," according to the *McGovern Report*, "is not why should we change our diet, but why not? What are the risks associated with eating less meat, less fat, less saturated fat, less cholesterol, less sugar, less salt, and more fruits, vegetables, unsaturated fat, and cereal products—especially whole-grain cereals? There are none that can be identified, and important benefits can be expected."[10]

The *McGovern Report* set forth a clear plan for Americans to increase their intake of fruits; starches such as whole grains, legumes, and root vegetables; nonstarchy vegetables such as broccoli, cauliflower, and green beans; and leafy greens like kale and lettuce. In addition to salt and simple sugars, the report suggested Americans reduce saturated fats, most notably meat, poultry, milk, butter, and cheese. It also stressed the urgency to act: "Ischemic heart disease, cancer, diabetes, and hypertension are the diseases that kill us. They are epidemic in our population. We cannot afford to temporize. We have an obligation to inform the public of the current state of knowledge and to assist the public in making the correct food choices. To do less is to avoid our responsibility."[11]

After 1968, death rates from heart disease decreased steadily, at an average rate of 3 percent per year, a direct result to the American public's change in diet and the country's seemingly mass smoking cessation.[12]

The truth was out, and I believed at that time that the United States and the world were on an unstoppable course to better health. Obviously, I was wrong, because the food industries went ballistic. Big Food was not going to repeat Big Tobacco's fate. A few months after the release of the *McGovern Report,* the beef and dairy businesses pushed back at a second Senate hearing, which resulted in a watered-down version of the *Dietary Goals,* with less emphasis on reducing meat and dairy products. The American Medical Association (AMA) also protested the *McGovern Report,* because it said that providing this basic knowledge on what we should eat might interfere with the medical doctor's right to prescribe, even though doctors then, as now, know essentially nothing about human nutrition.[13]

Even with this strong backlash from the industry, the effects of the *McGovern Report* were widespread and influential. In 1988, C. Everett Koop issued *The Surgeon General's Report on Nutrition and Health,* which, in echoing the *McGovern Report,* recommended a major increase in whole grains, vegetables, and fruits in our diet and an economy-shifting reduction in the consumption of meat and dairy products. As a result, the consumption of meat, milk products, and eggs did fall, albeit temporarily.

But these industries continued to fight back with every means at their disposal, including hiring lobbyists; purchasing medical and nutrition experts; launching huge advertising campaigns; educating schoolteachers, dietitians, medical doctors, and scientists; holding conferences for these professionals with speakers who favored, in return for big dollars, their products; hiring top-notch public-relation firms; and funding nutrition research supporting their sickening and fattening foods. The industries today essentially own the scientific studies, the journals they are published in, and the media to advertise their products.

Their success can be measured by the U.S. food availability data, which documents an increase in mean daily total energy intake, which jumped from 2,057 kilocalories in 1970 to 2,405 in 1990, 2,674 in 2008, and 3,770 in 2014.[14] We consume almost twice as much sugar, meat, poultry, dairy, eggs, and seafood today than we did in 1977, when the *McGovern Report* was issued. And it is no accident that the percentage of people suffering from overweight and obesity has doubled, and type 2 diabetes has more than tripled, during this same period.[15]

I have been in the general practice of medicine for nearly a half a century, thirty-nine years of which have been as a board-certified internist. Most of my practice has been focused on treating dietary diseases. Coupled with my experiences, national statistics tell me that nearly 70 percent of the population is overweight, with a staggering 38 percent now categorized as obese.[16] What's more, prediabetes affects half of our population, while 14 percent of the population has a high enough blood-sugar level to be diagnosed with type 2 diabetes.[17] By 2030, according to current projections, 44 percent of Americans will be obese—not overweight or heavy, but obese.[18] These figures are shocking, undeniable evidence that Big Food is still winning, while the men, women, and children of the United States are literally becoming casualties of the industries' unimpeded success.

The Current *Dietary Guidelines*

In addition to minimizing the dangers of cholesterol, the most recent *Dietary Guidelines for Americans 2015–2020* went out of its way to tell average Americans to pack as many nutrients, especially from meat, poultry, dairy, eggs, and fish, into their daily diet as possible, a laughable suggestion because Americans do not have nutrient-deficiency problems.[19]

If Americans don't have nutrient deficiencies, you may ask, then what are the problems? Simply put, Americans are suffering from overnutrition: they are overloaded with cholesterol, fat, protein, and calcium—from animal foods and vegetable oils, which the USDA so aggressively recommends as part of its dietary guidelines. Even when it's trying to help the American public, the USDA can't seem to get out of its own way. It can't get out of its own way because it trips over its strong political and financial ties to Big Food, overwhelmingly favoring in its guidelines the welfare of the meat, poultry, dairy, fish, and egg industries over the health and well-being of average Americans. At best, the USDA's stance on nutrition can be described as schizophrenic. At worst, it can be described as intentionally misleading and deadly.[20]

In advance of the USDA's recommendations, on January 6, 2016, I cofiled a lawsuit with the Physicians Committee for Responsible Medicine (PCRM) and other well-respected California-based physicians in the U.S. District Court for the Northern District of California against the USDA and the DHHS over their Dietary Guidelines Advisory Committee's position that "cholesterol is no longer a nutrient of concern for overconsumption."[21]

As physicians, we objected to this position on two grounds. The first is that cholesterol is very much a nutrient of concern, particularly in excessive quantities. Foods high in cholesterol, mainly meat, poultry, eggs, dairy products, and fish, can lead to obesity, heart disease (atherosclerosis), diabetes, inflammatory arthritis, and various intestinal disorders. The committee's language about cholesterol is largely based on a twenty-year attempt by the egg industry to change the public's image of eggs as a contributor to coronary artery disease (heart attacks), the number-one cause of death in America. Disregarding decades of independent basic research incriminating cholesterol consumption—"eating animals"—to accomplish their task, the USDA and DHHS instead relied on recent research that was orchestrated and funded by the egg and other livestock industries to communicate the innocence of eggs as a major cause of the multiple illnesses that plague millions of Americans.[22]

Second, my coplaintiffs and I argued in the injunction that the committee's claim that "cholesterol is no longer a nutrient of concern for overconsumption" interfered with our ability as physicians to accomplish our professional objectives and duties to keep our patients healthy and reverse dietary diseases.

Though our hearing for an injunction has yet to be heard, it may have already had an impact, albeit a minor one, on the USDA and the DHHS, which released the *Dietary Guidelines for Americans 2015–2020* with the following caveat about cholesterol consumption:

> The Key Recommendation from the 2010 Dietary Guidelines
> to limit consumption of dietary cholesterol to 300 mg per
> day is not included in the 2015 edition, but this change does

not suggest that dietary cholesterol is no longer important to consider when building healthy eating patterns. As recommended by the IOM (Institute of Medicine), individuals should eat as little dietary cholesterol as possible while consuming a healthy eating pattern. Strong evidence from mostly prospective cohort studies, but also randomized controlled trials, has shown that eating patterns that include lower intake of dietary cholesterol are associated with reduced risk of CVD (cardiovascular disease), and moderate evidence indicates that these eating patterns are associated with reduced risk of obesity.[23]

Eating "as little dietary cholesterol as possible" means following the Healthiest Diet on the Planet, since cholesterol is found in harmful amounts only in animal foods (meat, poultry, dairy, fish, and eggs), not plants.

Marketing Meat, Milk, and Disease

A marketing tactic widely used by Big Food is a method called "unique positioning." The objective is to cause a clear, unique, and advantageous position about their product to occupy consumers' minds. Focusing on a few unique qualities about a food and ignoring, or, worse yet, taking efforts to minimize harmful qualities found alongside these unique qualities, causes people to make food choices that can sicken themselves and their families.

For example, if I mention protein, you instinctively think of meat, poultry, and/or eggs. This is because the livestock industries have spent a lot of money making this connection for you. The truth is, however, that proteins are found in abundance in all natural foods, both plant and animal. No cases of protein deficiency have ever been reported on any natural diet, including a diet made from only plant foods.[24] "Protein deficiency" is a concern invented by the livestock industries to sell products. Never mentioned in the promotion of protein-packed food products is the abundance of calories, saturated fat, cholesterol, environmental chemicals, and microbes in them. In practical dietary terms, saturated fat is essentially synonymous with meat, poultry, dairy, and eggs. In addition, excess protein is a serious burden on the kidneys and liver, and excess animal protein causes calcium loss from the bones, resulting in osteoporosis and kidney stones.[25]

The same technique of "unique positioning" is used by the dairy industry. I say "calcium," and you think "milk." Yet no cases of calcium deficiency have ever been found in humans on any natural diet.[26] (You may be thinking osteoporosis is caused by lack of calcium, but excess animal protein is the real primary dietary culprit.) The fish industries have fooled you into believing that fish is the best source of essential fats. Thus, a "unique position" is created by these industries so you will buy their fish to get your omega-3 fats. The truth is, only plants can make these essential fats. The fish got their omega-3s from eating algae and seaweed. Why not go directly to the source? Plants!

What chance, then, do consumers have of attaining good health when the meat, poultry, fish, dairy, and egg industries advertise their products as the ideal, practical, and only means to get these three essential nutrients—protein, calcium, and omega-3 fats? Very little. The only way to counter misinformation and deception is with sound information and unimpeachable scientific research.

The Healthiest Solution Is Known

For each and every animal there is a diet that provides optimal health. That diet contains an ideal mixture of fuels from protein, fat, and sugars (carbohydrates) along with vitamins, minerals, and other nutrients to meet a particular animal's needs. Cats, for instance, are carnivores; they thrive on the flesh of other animals. They have taste buds on their tongue for proteins, but none for sugars (carbohydrates).[27] Thus, the bulk of their fuel comes from protein and fat and almost none from sugars. Meanwhile, hippopotamuses thrive on broadleaf plants; most of their calories come from natural sugars and very few from fat. Dogs are omnivores, which means they can survive well on a wide variety of foods from the plant and animal kingdoms and obtain energy efficiently from all three classes of fuels.

Based on the foods you see your friends and family eat, you would guess the digestion processes and nutritional needs of people were more akin to those of dogs: eating anything and everything. Even so, many foods people eat daily—from cotton candy to pork rinds—are so nutritionally worthless, that you would never threaten your pet's health with them.

Fortunately, human beings, as survivors, are able to live at the extremes of nutrition. The Eskimos, for instance, eat an all-meat diet for most of the year,[28] a diet mimicked these days by the low-carb diets ("bacon, butter, and Brie") made famous by Dr. Robert Atkins. At the other extreme is the medically based diet of white rice, fruit, fruit juice, and table sugar developed by Walter Kempner, M.D., and used at Duke University for seven decades to heal people with arthritis, type 2 diabetes, heart disease, hypertension, kidney disease, and obesity.[29] Almost everyone eats in between these extremes. Most healthy people eat a "well-balanced diet," which they believe keeps them free of life-threatening deficiencies of protein and calcium and the most recently recognized deficiency, that of omega-3 fats. But eating between the extremes does not make a healthy diet. Just the opposite.

The Standard American Diet (SAD) has changed little in the last forty years, and the health and obesity crisis is clear evidence that this is not the way forward. Here's a reasonable breakdown of the percentages of the foods found in the Standard American Diet:

- 70 percent meat and dairy products

- 20 percent simple sugars and refined starches

- 5 percent fruit

- 5 percent nonstarchy vegetables

This is 100 percent a formula for weight gain, poor daily health, and a significant increased risk for obesity, type 2 diabetes, heart disease, and cancer. This, as we've already seen, is a losing formula when it comes to health and longevity.

The Healthiest Diet on the Planet, on the other hand, offers a scientifically based alternative that immediately helps you lose weight, feel better, protects you against life-threatening disease, and even reverses most common chronic diseases. This is a simple and proven formula that I have been sharing with my patients for four decades, one that always yields life-changing results. These are the very foods that we as humans are designed to eat, these are the foods we crave,

Carbohydrates: A Closer Look

Carbohydrates are made by plants and stored in their leaves, stems, roots, flowers, and fruits. Plant foods contain both simple and complex carbohydrates in various amounts. Fruits often contain 90 percent of their calories as carbohydrates, and most are the sweet-tasting simple sugars, such as glucose and fructose. Green and yellow vegetables store most of their calories as complex carbohydrates, but since they contain very few total calories, the amount of energy they provide in the diet is small. The best sources of carbohydrates are whole grains (rice and corn), whole-grain flours (barley, corn, rice, wheat, and rye as well as whole-grain pastas made from them, such as wheat and soba noodles), tubers (potatoes, sweet potatoes, and yams), legumes (beans, lentils, and peas), and winter squashes (acorn and Hubbard)—all of which contain sufficient quantities of energy to fuel your daily needs from complex carbohydrates and thus are known as starches. Rice, corn, and other grains as well as potatoes typically store about 80 percent of their calories in the form of starch. Beans, peas, and lentils are approximately 70 percent starch.

Carbohydrates are the preferred source of energy for our tissues, and all of the cells in our bodies can use carbohydrates for energy. The carbohydrate glucose is essential for the brain (about 140 grams a day are utilized). However, under unusual circumstances, such as when someone is starving to death or following a low-carb diet for long periods, the brain can adapt to burn ketones from fats. Not surprisingly, brain function in people has been found to be impaired when the body burns ketones rather than glucose.[30] There is also concern that long-term adherence to a low-carb (ketone-producing) diet may cause permanent damage to the developing brain.[31] Certain tissues such as red blood cells and some of the kidney cells can only burn glucose. Fortunately, during carbohydrate deprivation the body will convert protein into glucose, through a process known as gluconeogenesis, to keep blood and kidney cells alive.

We typically store 2 pounds of carbohydrate in our muscles and liver as glycogen (as branched chains of sugars). These reserves are immediately available to supply the brain and other carbohydrate-burning tissues during long periods between meals. They also serve to provide a steady supply of fuel for athletes during endurance events.

You've probably heard that marathon runners and other endurance athletes "load up" on carbohydrates before an event in order to store energy-providing fuel for the long race. They do this because they want to win. Loading up on carbohydrates several times a day will also give you the energy to race through your busy life.

The only food from animals in which carbohydrates are found in significant amounts is their milk, which contains a simple sugar called lactose, but lactose can't be digested by most adults and consequently can cause assorted signs and symptoms of indigestion, such as diarrhea, stomach cramps, and painful amounts of gas.

In general, Americans eat far too few calories from carbohydrates—only about 40 percent. To make things worse, the kinds of carbohydrates eaten most commonly are "empty calories" in the form of white sugar, corn syrup, and fructose. The Healthiest Diet on the Planet encourages you to consume 70 to 90 percent of your calories from starches (barley, beans, corn, potatoes, sweet potatoes, rice, wheat, etc.) and the remainder from other vegetables and fruits.

these are the foods that unbiased studies have proved to be the most health promoting.

Although human beings can survive on many different varieties of food, in order to function, feel, and look our best, we must lean heavily on our biological design as herbivores, plant eaters. But not just any plants. We are starch eaters, also referred to as starchivores or starchitarians.[32] Starches are plant parts that store an abundance of energy, otherwise known as carbohydrates, to power our rocket-building brains and to sustain muscles that can run for days without stopping. That special fuel is sugar, which is stored as long chains in starchy plant parts often referred to as complex carbohydrates. Starches that grow underground, such as potatoes and sweet potatoes, are so nutritionally complete that a person can live in excellent health on these foods alone.[33] Starches provide an abundance of protein, vitamins, minerals, and dietary fiber, with just enough essential fat to meet all of our dietary needs. Grains and legumes, however, need a little help from fruits, like oranges, and green or yellow vegetables, like broccoli, in order to provide adequate vitamin A and C.

The most important evidence supporting my claim that the natural human diet is based on starches is a simple observation that you can easily validate for yourself: all large populations of trim, healthy, athletic, war-fighting people, throughout verifiable human history, have obtained the bulk of their calories from starch.[34] Examples of once-thriving people include Japanese, Chinese, and other Asians, who ate sweet potatoes, buckwheat, and/or rice; Incas, in South America, who ate potatoes; Mayans and Aztecs, in Central America, who ate corn; and Egyptians, in the Middle East, who ate wheat. There have been only a few small isolated populations of primitive people, such as the Arctic Inuit Eskimos, living at the extremes of the environment who have eaten otherwise. Therefore, scientific written documentation of what people have eaten over the past thirteen thousand years convincingly supports my claim. Archaeological evidence shows we have been starch eaters for more than a hundred thousand years. Evidence of pre–*Homo sapiens* dates plant eating to 2.6 million years ago for humanoids.[35]

The Truth about Protein

Any natural diet, as long as it contains a sufficient amount of calories, will always—I repeat, always—fulfill your body's need for protein. In fact, there has never been a single case of protein deficiency reported in the world that resulted from any natural diet with a sufficient number of calories.[36] Kwashiorkor, a severe protein deficiency, only occurs as a result of extreme starvation (in which case all nutrients are deficient).[37] Isolated protein deficiency caused by avoiding animal-derived foods is a fallacy. Plants also provide all of the essential amino acids that make up these proteins in order to meet our needs.[38]

Meanwhile, billions of people are suffering and dying because they're eating too much protein. Respected researchers find that those hunter-gatherer populations that have based their diets on meat, such as the Inuits (Eskimos), suffer from heart disease and other forms of atherosclerosis, while hunter-gatherers who have based their diets on plant foods (starches) are free of these diseases.[39] Also epidemic among the meat- and fish-consuming hunter-gatherers, like the Eskimos, is osteoporosis.[40]

Eating excess high-protein, animal-derived foods in addition contributes to our most common diseases for many well-established reasons, including the indisputable facts that they are high in cholesterol, most are high in fat, and they contain no dietary fiber or digestible carbohydrates. They are also filthy with disease-causing microbes (including, but not limited to, mad cow prions; listeria, E. coli, and salmonella bacteria; and leukemia viruses) and contain the highest levels of poisonous environmental chemicals found in the food chain.[41]

Protein accelerates growth for good and bad. Meat and dairy products stimulate growth by various mechanisms, which include raising levels of insulin-like growth factor-1 (IGF-1).[42] Resembling insulin in its chemical structure, IGF-1 accelerates the rate of growth of normal and diseased tissues, bone, and cancer, respectively. Activities from this hormone also accelerate aging. Mice with lower levels of IGF-1, according to numerous experiments, live 40 percent longer than mice with normal levels of IGF-1.[43] What's more, as these mice get older, they not only look younger, but, more importantly, they resist diseases and chronic ailments of the aging process. They have good eyes, healthy joints, high-functioning brains, and sustained immunity. Presently, researchers believe our best hope for increasing longevity is by lowering IGF-1 activity.

All animal foods—cow's milk, in particular—raise IGF-1 levels in humans.[44] The purpose of cow's milk is to accelerate the growth of a cow from 60 to 600 pounds. Because protein promotes growth, a diet high in protein, regardless of the source, automatically raises IGF-1 levels. A good example of this effect by vegetable protein is seen with the isolated soy protein used in synthetic foods, from candy bars to burgers, which is an even more powerful promoter of IGF-1 than cow's milk.[45]

Foods That Raise IGF-1
Protein in general
Isolated soy protein
Milk
Meat
Poultry
Fish
Seafood[46]

The benefits of lowering your IGF-1 activity, through something as simple as making sensible food choices, can be documented in people. A study of 292 British women ages twenty to seventy years found that the serum IGF-1 activity was 13 percent lower in the 92 women who followed a vegan diet compared to the level in the 99 meat eaters and 101 lacto-ovo-vegetarians.[47] Similar effects have been found in men following vegan diets.[48]

High Cholesterol Is a Sign of Poor Health

Another danger in eating animal-derived food, whether it's tuna or turkey, is the risk of higher cholesterol. You just read that the Dietary Guidelines Advisory Committee wanted to argue that cholesterol was "no longer a nutrient of concern for overconsumption," but yet the evidence that dietary cholesterol is poisonous is overwhelming and growing. A letter from the *American Journal of Clinical Nutrition* summarizes the research: "As shown in thousands of animal experiments in mammals and birds, including nonhuman primates, the addition of cholesterol to their usual diet is virtually a requirement for the production of atherosclerosis. Even the addition of small amounts of cholesterol to the diet of rabbits, chickens, and monkeys—resulting in little or no increase in blood cholesterol—produces atherosclerosis in the long term nonetheless."[49] Human studies have confirmed the causative relationship between eating cholesterol-containing animal food and heart disease and strokes.[50]

Of all the foods commonly consumed as part of the rich Western diet, eggs contain the highest concentrations of cholesterol. Eggs contain eight times more cholesterol than beef (see box below). Traditionally, in scientific studies on humans, eggs have been used as the source to demonstrate the adverse effects of cholesterol on our health and our heart arteries. In response, the egg industry has purposely misled the public and its practicing physicians about the

The Richest Sources of Cholesterol

FOOD	MG/100 CALORIES
Whole Eggs	272
Lobster	73
Salmon	41
Chicken	37
Beef	33
All Plant Foods	0

harmful effects of eggs, which are poisonous when consumed in the high amounts typical of American diets.

The egg industry provides a timely example of how money can buy scientific nutritional information that can be detrimental to the public's health. In my 1983 national best-selling book *The McDougall Plan,* I revealed the dirty tricks the egg industry has used to get Americans to eat more eggs since the late 1970s. More than three decades ago, I noted that of the six studies in the medical literature that fail to demonstrate a significant rise in blood cholesterol level with the consumption of whole eggs, three were paid for by the American Egg Board, one by the Missouri Egg Merchandising Council, and one by the Egg Program of the California Department of Agriculture; support for the sixth paper was not identified.

In contrast, well-designed studies by investigators independent of the food industry clearly demonstrate the detrimental effects of eggs on blood-cholesterol levels. The actual impact of eating eggs is seen when people who eat little cholesterol are fed eggs. When seventeen lactovegetarian college students (consuming 97 milligrams of cholesterol daily) were fed one extra-large egg daily for three weeks, their LDL ("bad") cholesterol increased by 12 percent.[51] I have written extensively about the research showing that including eggs in your diet is an unwise decision.[52]

Writing in the *American Journal of Clinical Nutrition* in 1998, Jeremiah Stamler, M.D., the chairman of the Department of Preventive Medicine of the Feinberg School of Medicine (Northwestern University), commented:

> It is a reasonable inference that the sizable decline in per capita egg consumption in the United States in recent

Common Examples of Starches, Nonstarchy Vegetables, and Fruits

Starches

Starches are defined as foods that contain adequate amounts of readily available calories in the form of starch molecules.

Whole Grains

Barley, bulgur (cracked wheat), buckwheat, millet, oats, rice, rye, triticale, wheat berries

Legumes

Beans: adzuke (azuki), black, garbanzo, great northern, kidney, lima, mung, navy, pink, pinto, soy, white

Peas: black-eyed, split green, split yellow

Lentils: brown, green, red

Starchy Vegetables

Parsnips, potatoes, salsify, sweet potatoes, winter squashes (acorn, banana, butternut, Hubbard), yams

Nonstarchy Vegetables

Vegetables are defined as plants or plant parts that are too low in calorie content to form the center of a meal. However, they do provide valuable contributions of vitamins, minerals, fiber, water, essential fat, protein, and other plant (phyto-) nutrients, to say nothing of the aroma, flavor, color, and variety in texture they can bring to your meal.

Summer Squash: chayote, crook-neck, scalloped cocozelle, straight-neck, zucchini

Roots: beet, carrots, Jerusalem artichokes, onion, radish, turnip

Pods: Chinese pea, green bean, yellow (wax) bean

Mushrooms: button, shiitake, straw, winter

Flowers: artichoke, broccoli, Brussels sprouts, cauliflower

Leaves: cabbage, chard, kale, lettuce, spinach

Stalks: asparagus, celery, rhubarb

Fruitlike: cucumber, eggplant, tomato

Fruits

Fruit is a pleasing addition to the basic starch-centered meal or can be consumed as dessert or as a snack between meals.

Citrus: grapefruit, lemon, lime, orange, tangerine

Noncitrus: apple, avocado, banana, cantaloupe, cherry, cucumber, grape, guava, honeydew, kiwi, lychee, mango, nectarine, olive, papaya, passion fruit, peach, pear, pineapple, plum, strawberry, tomato, watermelon

Note: Tomatoes, cucumbers, avocados, and olives are actually fruits, even though many people think of them as vegetables. Avocados and olives have a very high fat content, and dried fruits provide a very high concentration of simple sugar calories. Initially, these are to be avoided in your diet, especially if you are trying to lose weight.

decades, and hence in per capita total cholesterol intake, has been one important component of the improved dietary patterns leading to a fall in mean serum cholesterol concentration in the adult population from ~ 6.08 mmol/L (235 mg/dL) in the 1950s to ~ 5.30 mmol/L (205 mg/dL) in the 1990s, and to the concomitant sustained marked reductions in mortality rates from CHD [coronary heart disease], all cardiovascular diseases, and all causes.[53]

Between 1970 and 1995 annual consumption decreased from 310 to 235 eggs per person.[54] But, in the years since, annual consumption has shot back up to about 260 eggs per person.

The purpose of a hen's egg is to provide all the materials necessary to develop the one cell created by the joining of a cock's sperm with a hen's ovum into a complete chick with feathers, a beak, two eyeballs, two wings, two legs, and a tail. This miraculous growth and development is supported by a 1.5-ounce package of ingredients, the hen's egg, jam-packed with proteins, fats, cholesterol, vitamins, and minerals. The hen's egg has been called "one of nature's most nutritious creations"—for growing chicks.

Indeed, an egg is the richest of all foods—and far too much of a "good thing" for people. The components of a cooked egg are completely absorbed through our intestines. As a result, this highly concentrated food, recommended by the *Dietary Guidelines for Americans 2015–2020,* provides too much cholesterol, fat, and protein for our body to process safely. The penalties are heart disease, obesity, osteoporosis, and type 2 diabetes, to name a few epidemic sicknesses promoted by egg consumption.

The Healthiest Diet on the Planet

By nature we are designed to enjoy and thrive on starches. Bread is known as "the staff of life." Noodle dishes are referred to as "comfort food." The Japanese have cultivated rice for over two thousand years as their principal crop. The fundamental importance of rice to the Japanese people is reflected by the fact that rice was once used as currency and the formal Japanese word for "cooked rice" (*gohan*) also means "meal." The literal meaning of "breakfast" (*asa gohan*), for example, is "morning rice." In China the word for "rice" is also the word for "food." The Chinese say, "A meal without rice is like a beautiful woman with only one eye." Instead of the typical greeting, "How are you?" the Chinese ask, "Have you had your rice today?" In India, rice is the first food a new bride offers her husband. In Indonesia, no girl can be considered for marriage until she can skillfully prepare rice.

This is not a new diet. Until a century ago almost every person on earth ate a starch-based diet (excluding the aristocracy). Their foods were mostly—say 90 percent—starches, with some fruits and green and yellow vegetables added in when they were in season. Meat, poultry, dairy foods, eggs, fish, seafood, cookies, pies, and candies were eaten only occasionally, served as delicacies. As a result, people were trim, strong, and free of the diseases common in people living today. The exceptions were the kings, queens, pharaohs, priests, and other aristocrats, who ate rich foods daily, at every meal like Americans, and in the process developed obesity, diabetes, atherosclerosis, gout, and tooth decay as well as all of the other chronic dietary diseases found in modern men, women, and children.

It should come as no surprise, then, that starches will also make up to 90 percent of your daily calories while following the Healthiest Diet on the Planet. The remainder of the diet consists of nonstarchy plant parts, such as kale, broccoli, asparagus, and cauliflower. Plus, you should enjoy some fruits.

Here is a breakdown of the percentages of the foods on the Healthiest Diet on the Planet:

- 70 to 90 percent starch (pasta, potatoes, rice, bread)

- 10 to 20 percent nonstarchy vegetables

- 5 to 10 percent fruit

- 0 percent meat, poultry, fish, eggs, dairy, and vegetable oils

As you can see, I am asking you to remove meat, poultry, dairy, eggs, and fish (all animal foods) and vegetable oils from your diet entirely. The Healthiest Diet on the Planet consists of the foods that will help you lose weight, stay trim, feel fit, look attractive, perform athletically, fight off disease, and live longer and happier. These foods also happen to be foods you love and naturally crave, including those foods that we are commonly told to avoid—bread, pasta, pizza, potatoes, rice, and even pancakes, to name just a few of the wonderful options you'll enjoy on the Healthiest Diet on the Planet.

I would like to add that this is not "an all or nothing" recommendation. I must, however, teach you the best I know, and then you will do the best you can. Results are usually proportional to the changes you make, but some conditions, such as inflammatory arthritis, require strict adherence to the program.

My Own Research

After caring for more than six thousand patients in a live-in residential setting, I can tell you all of them have benefited from a change to the Healthiest Diet on the Planet. In October 2014 the *Nutrition Journal* published my study looking at the results of 1,615 people following the Healthiest Diet on the Planet.[55] (No patients were excluded from the study.) Titled "Effects of 7 Days on an Ad Libitum Low-Fat Vegan Diet: The McDougall Program Cohort," this important scientific research documented the effects of eating a low-fat (less than 10 percent of calories from fat), high-carbohydrate (about 80 percent of calories from carbs), moderate-sodium, purely plant-based diet, enjoyed to the full satisfaction of the appetite for seven days, on the biomarkers of cardiovascular disease and type 2 diabetes. ("Ad libitum," by the way, means you can eat as much as you want.)

The median weight loss of the group was 3.1 pounds (1.4 kg). The median decrease in total cholesterol was 22 mg/dL (.6 IU). Even though most blood pressure and diabetic medications were reduced or discontinued in the beginning, systolic blood pressure (top number) decreased by 8 mmHg, diastolic blood pressure by 4 mmHg, and blood glucose by 3 mg/dL on average. (Medication reductions were made in approximately 90 percent of patients who were taking these drugs at the beginning of the program.) Based on these changes in numbers (risk factors), for patients whose risk of a cardiovascular event within ten years was over 7.5 percent at baseline, the risk dropped to 5.5 percent in only seven days.

These are average changes; those who started out sicker got even more dramatic results. When the cholesterol began at over 240 mg/dL the fall in seven days was on average 39 mg/dL. If the blood pressure was initially high (140/90 mmHg or greater), then the average reduction was 18/11 mmHg, and the blood pressure medication was discontinued in most cases. The people in the study attended my ten-day, live-in program in Santa Rosa, California, where they experienced the same education and edification you will receive throughout this book. They also ate the same kinds of foods you will find reflected in the recipes in this book. Which means you can expect the same results when you follow the Healthiest Diet on the Planet as outlined in these pages.

What was not reported in the publication about my live-in program using the Healthiest Diet on the Planet at my clinic, however, was the fact that within twenty-four hours most people found relief from constipation, indigestion, gastroesophageal reflux disease (GERD), oily skin, fatigue, and much more. Within four months most chronic problems from food poisoning such as inflammatory arthritis, chest pains (angina), skin diseases, and chronic head and body aches were a matter of history.

On my plan, the average weight loss in those who need to lose is about 8 to 16 pounds a month without restriction of the amount of food eaten. Heavier people lose quicker. Exercise can be helpful, but is not required for losing excess body fat. It is the high-carbohydrate, high-fiber, and very low-fat composition of the starches that changes the body. This is a cost-free, side effect–free treatment.

You might argue that these are merely short-term results and cannot be sustained. However, we have scientific documentation to the contrary. Between 2009 and 2013 the Neurology Department of the Oregon Health & Science University (OHSU), the medical school in Portland, Oregon, independently compared twenty-nine patients who went through my ten-day live-in program and continued the plan in varying degrees with a control group of a similar number who did not follow the program over a yearlong period.[56] The study design, known as a randomized, rater-blinded, controlled trial, was of the highest scientific quality. The initial intention of the study was to determine the safety and feasibility of the diet for people with multiple sclerosis (MS). The results were astonishing.

The intervention group, or those going through my residential program in Santa Rosa, California, following the Healthiest Diet on the Planet, reduced their dietary fat consumption as a percent of total calories from 40 to 15 and maintained that level for one year. (The control group remained at 40 percent of their calories from fat for a year.) We estimate from our food-frequency questionnaire data that 85 percent of the diet group followed the program 100 percent of the time for the study period of one year. In other words, they permanently changed their diet. At the end of a year they also attained and maintained on average a 19.1 pound (8.7 kg) weight loss and on average a 19 mg/dL (0.5 IU) reduction in cholesterol. These fabulous numbers were seen in people who are younger (forty-one years) than our average patients (fifty-eight years). Furthermore, these people were not primarily interested in losing weight and lowering cholesterol; they were focused on their multiple sclerosis. People following the Healthiest Diet on the Planet who make the change primarily for weight and cholesterol problems should expect either the same or even more dramatic permanent results.

Too Good to Be True?

Although these results might seem too good to be true, the Healthiest Diet on the Planet offers a scientifically based alternative that immediately helps you lose weight, feel better, protect yourself against life-threatening medical problems, and reverse common diseases. This is a simple and proven formula that I have been sharing with patients for four decades. The Healthiest Diet on the Planet continues to yield life-changing results. Its success is the result of its simplicity; it is made up of the very foods we as humans are designed to eat. The Healthiest Diet on the Planet is made up of the very foods we crave. The Healthiest Diet on the Planet is made up of the very foods that science has shown to promote longevity.

Observing the health and longevity of people who eat better than Americans provides clues to the potential gains from reducing chronic diseases. As I introduced above, the Japanese people, who eat a diet based on starches (rice and vegetables) with little meat and no dairy products, have an average life-span of 85.6 years for women and 78.6 years for men—four to five years longer than people following the American diet.[57] Vegetarian Seventh-Day Adventists do even better: women live on average to 88.6 and men to 85.3.[58] In fact, a direct comparison with other white Californians found vegetarian Adventists live an average of ten years longer. However, these vigorous Adventist vegetarians still include way too much dairy, eggs, soy protein, and vegetable oils in their diets to achieve the full potential of human longevity—leaving people who are fully informed the opportunity to add even a few more "good" years.

The November 2005 issue of *National Geographic* magazine

published an excellent article, "The Secrets of Living Longer."[59] It reported on three groups of long-lived people from Okinawa, Japan; Sardinia, Italy; and Loma Linda, California—all of whom followed a plant-based diet. Nicoya, Costa Rica, and Icaria, Greece, have recently been added to the list of the locations of the longest-lived and healthiest people on the planet. Collectively, these countries are often referred to as the "blue zones." Inhabitants of these isolated regions consume diets based on locally grown starches and live to the age of one hundred at rates ten times higher than the average American.

The world has changed greatly over the past thirty-five years. More than 90 percent of the world's rice is produced and consumed by people living in the Far East.[60] However, as the wealth of people in this part of the world has increased, the consumption of meat and dairy foods and vegetable oils has more than doubled over the past thirty-five years, while the consumption of rice per capita has decreased.[61] To no one's surprise, the health of people worldwide has deteriorated during this same period, with alarming, near epidemic increases in obesity, heart disease, and type 2 diabetes.[62]

Such findings provide a timely and potent counterargument to the *Journal of the American Medical Association*'s opinion piece calling for the removal of an upper limit on the intake of total dietary fat and applauding the "elimination of dietary cholesterol as a 'nutrient of concern'" for the *Dietary Guidelines for Americans 2015–2020*.[63]

The fundamental message I am sharing with you is that *it's the food*. The results are yours for the taking with no risk, costs, or side effects. Is it worth it? Of course it is!

I love life so much I would happily eat a plateful of cardboard to spend another afternoon windsurfing, one more hour playing with any of my seven grandchildren, or one more evening with my wife,

Mary. About to enter my seventh decade of life, I can hardly believe how young and healthy I feel. As long as I am functional, comfortable, and content, I want to live to be a hundred too.

Fortunately, I don't have to eat cardboard to achieve a long life. Nor do I have to sacrifice full satisfaction of my appetite or the enjoyment of my meals in favor of health. And neither do you. By *its natural composition,* the Healthiest Diet on the Planet controls the intake of calories, fat, protein, carbohydrate, vitamins, and minerals effortlessly without ever causing hunger. Now *that* is what I call a program you can live with for years and years, well into your golden age.

2

The McDougall Story

was born and raised in the suburbs of Detroit. Like any good midwesterner, my mother fed me meat and dairy, the foods she had been taught were the most nutritious. Despite my mother's best intentions, these foods caused me serious health problems throughout my childhood and high-school years: painful constipation, oily skin, terrible acne on my face, and poor endurance on the athletic field. In 1965, when I went to college at age eighteen at Michigan State University, I suffered a major stroke, a condition that today strikes about a thousand teenagers annually in the United States. No doubt the cafeteria foods served at my college dormitory provided the final assaults to my arteries.

An angiogram showed a blockage in a small but critical artery in the right side of my brain (a lacunar infarct). The stroke caused complete paralysis of the entire left side of my body. It took me two weeks before I was able to move my left thumb one-quarter of an inch—an accomplishment that in my estimation meant it was time to discharge myself from Grace Hospital in downtown Detroit. After several months, I recovered about 60 percent of my strength and coordination. I still walk with a noticeable limp today, fifty years later.

My cafeteria diet at Snyder Hall dormitory at Michigan State was the standard animal-based diet, and I was free to eat all I wanted. It was not unusual for me to go back for thirds of bacon and eggs for breakfast, consume three beef hamburgers for lunch, and down a plate load of pork chops for dinner. And most of my male friends at college did the same.

Four years later, after entering the College of Human Medicine (medical school) at Michigan State University, I weighed about 230 pounds (my maximum weight). Hospitals provided medical students during their training with free food in the dining room. I became so heavy by age twenty-two that even my own mother called me fat. Due to my diet of eggs for breakfast, bologna sandwiches for lunch, and hot dogs, hamburgers, and pizza for dinner, I also had a cholesterol level of 338 mg/dL (still considered "normal" because elevated cholesterol at that time was 350 mg/dL or higher).

In the summer of 1971 I met my lifelong partner, Mary, and almost a year later we moved to Hawaii, where, at twenty-five, I began my postgraduate training at the Queen's Medical Center in Honolulu. There, the stomach pains that I had had for most of my life became so intense that they often forced me to curl up in bed with cramps after dinner. Finally, at Mary's insistence, I consulted a doctor. Unfortunately, because I was in the middle of my monthlong surgery rotation, the only opinion I got was from a surgeon, who suggested I undergo an exploratory abdominal procedure—that same afternoon!

Without asking me a single question about my diet, which included three chili dogs before bed most nights, the surgeon cut me open and removed a perfectly healthy appendix. My stomach pains never fully went away, but, like all other medical professionals I knew, I never once questioned the wisdom of eating a diet heavy in meat and dairy products. Little did I know that if I didn't change what and how I ate, I was headed for a short adult life of obesity, type 2 diabetes, heart disease, and a host of other illnesses, including prostate cancer and, most likely, a second stroke, which could have proven fatal.

Initial Insights

The turning point came soon after I finished my internship at the Queen's Medical Center. My first job was as a family practitioner caring for approximately five thousand workers at the Hamakua Sugar Plantation on the Big Island of Hawaii. I was twenty-six years old. As I was one of only four doctors practicing in the countryside, my responsibilities were unusually broad. I attended to life from beginning to end—delivering babies, repairing injuries, refilling monthly prescriptions, providing hospital care, and pronouncing people dead. As a result, I became a very experienced doctor, and, I am happy to report, most of my patients fared well.

My patient population consisted mostly of first-, second-, third-, and fourth-generation Japanese, Chinese, Koreans, and Filipinos. In this multigenerational mix of patients, I began to observe distinct patterns. Those in the first generation were always trim, usually active into their eighties and nineties, and never suffered from constipation, hemorrhoids, ulcers, diabetes, heart disease, multiple sclerosis, breast cancer, prostate cancer, or colon cancer, the most common illnesses in most Western populations. Their children and grandchildren, however, did. What was the difference?

Only one fundamental factor could account for the increasing gap between the excellent health of the first generation and the progressively deteriorating health of subsequent generations. That factor was diet. My first-generation patients had remained faithful to their native starch-based diet, which featured primarily white rice with the addition of fruits and vegetables. (We recommend whole-grain brown rice, but billions of people have thrived, free of obesity and Western diseases, on refined white rice.) Their American-born offspring, however, incorporated more rich Western foods into their diets, while cutting back on starches, fruits, and vegetables. As a result, they gained weight and became sicker.

I noticed this trend most strikingly in the Filipino population, specifically the older Filipino men with young wives and young children. After saving for years and then retiring, single men traveled to the Philippines in search of a young bride. In my office every day I witnessed what can best be described as the miracle of men in their seventies and eighties starting new families, demonstrating prowess (by what can only be described as "natural Viagra") that many American men can only fantasize about after their forties. In addition to siring healthy and beautiful children, my septuagenarian Filipino men expected to see their young children grow into adults, and they did. This virility and optimism resulted from their diet.

And yet I could rarely convince my younger patients to follow their parents' and grandparents' examples. Eventually, prescribing pill after pill to treat patients with chronic diseases, such as obesity, diabetes, hypertension, arthritis, heart disease, and life-threatening cancers, left me feeling incompetent and inadequate. My patients with chronic diseases never became well under my care.

It was becoming impossible for me to practice medicine the way I'd been taught. I had held two basic beliefs since childhood. The first was that as we age, we naturally become fatter and sicker. The second was that a "well-balanced" American-type diet was best. But my newfound knowledge about nutrition and health from my sugar-plantation experience was calling those beliefs into question. I had seen evidence that a starch-based diet allowed people to live longer and healthier lives. As a result, I began to adopt the eating habits of my healthiest elder patients and subsequently lost 40 pounds (I went from about 190 to 150 pounds). (Since then I have varied from 150 to 170 pounds. I am currently below 150 pounds at six feet tall. The change has depended upon how strictly I have adhered to what I know to be the Healthiest Diet on the Planet.)

Further Study: Six Mentors

After three years of general practice, Mary and I returned to Oahu, with our two children in tow, so I could learn how to become a more effective doctor. (We had our third child on Oahu in 1982.) For the next two years, I studied at the John A. Burn's School of Medicine at the University of Hawaii, before becoming a board-certified internal-medicine specialist. One great fortune of mine was the discovery of the Hawaii State Medical Library, on the grounds of the Queen's Medical Center, filled with thousands of scientific reports confirming the observations I had made while being a sugar-plantation physician. In 1978, a year after the Select Committee on Nutrition and Human Needs released the *McGovern Report*, I established a small general practice. The report was music to my ears, inspiring me to investigate further.

Reading through the scientific journals at the library, I learned that many other doctors and scientists before me had made similar discoveries. Diets featuring common starches, particularly beans, corn, potatoes, rice, and/or wheat, resulted in robust health, while meat, dairy, and vegetable oils destroyed people's physical condition. But I also discovered an even more important breakthrough. Once people stopped eating the foods that made them sick, they recovered. The message was something akin to, "Stop throwing gasoline on a fire." Scientific researchers described weight loss and relief from chronic chest pains (angina), headaches, and arthritis as well as the reversal of kidney disease, heart failure, type 2 diabetes, and many more physical ailments and conditions. Volumes of research written over the previous fifty years showed me how to cure my patients with one simple solution: a starch-based diet as presented in the Healthiest Diet on the Planet.

Dusty journals stacked on the library shelves led me to six mentors whose work has served as the foundation for my own. Denis Burkitt (1911–1993), medical doctor and surgeon, taught me about the importance of dietary fiber (indigestible carbohydrates present in plants) as well as the broader concept of a proper diet based on unrefined starches, green and yellow vegetables, fruits, and a limited amount of meat and dairy products.[1] He served for seventeen years as head of the governmental health services of Uganda, where he witnessed more than ten million people flourishing on grains and tubers, eating almost no meats, dairy products, or processed foods. These people had no obesity, heart disease, constipation, gallstones, hemorrhoids, multiple sclerosis, diabetes, or cancers of the breast, colon, or prostate. Before learning about Dr. Burkitt's revolutionary ideas, I foolishly believed that common chronic diseases were unsolvable mysteries, perhaps a product of viral infections or genetic mishaps. Being a doctor, I started to realize that this might mean more than treating the signs and symptoms of my suffering patients with pills and surgeries. Common diseases could be prevented, possibly cured, by eating simple, inexpensive foods—something I had recognized in my firsthand observations at the sugar plantation.

Meanwhile Russell Henry Chittenden (1856–1943) and William Rose (1887–1985) showed me the fallacy of protein deficiency.[2] My research in the library also led me to pioneer medical doctors Roy Swank (1909–2008)[3] and Walter Kempner (1903–1997),[4] who completely upended my understanding of nutrition, showing that diet therapy could work wonders on chronic and acute illnesses alike, from hypertension and fatigue to heart disease and—amazingly, thanks to Roy Swank, who later endorsed my starch-based protocol—multiple sclerosis, an autoimmune disease that attacks the tissues of the brain and spinal cord.

Around this same time, Nathan Pritikin (1915–1985) published his seminal Pritikin Program, which still serves as the foundation of much of my work. With his straight-from-nature, no-processed-foods protocol, Nathan Pritikin made public the kind of diet therapy I was just beginning to practice.[5] I first met Mr. Pritikin in May of 1979, during his visit to the island of Oahu, Hawaii. I invited him to my humble tract home in Kailua for dinner. Mary served him and his wife, Ilene, a simple meal of whole-grain bread, pasta, red sauce, and confetti rice salad. Peach pie was our dessert. He said he liked the meal a lot. Before he left, he autographed a copy of his new book, *The Pritikin Program for Diet & Exercise*.

On his next visit to Oahu three years later, Mr. Pritikin and I spent two days together. I was able to have him substitute for a scheduled speaker at the regular early-morning doctors' conference at Straub Clinic & Hospital. He was well received, except for one rude physician. I thought this doctor might have felt threatened by a non–medically trained person trying to teach him about curing patients with food. The next morning, I arranged for a special breakfast meeting in his honor with the medical staff and medical students at the Queen's Medical Center. Only two doctors attended. One shoveled greasy bacon and eggs into his mouth. Neither seemed interested in this physically small man whose big idea was to wipe out heart disease.

That evening we held a potluck dinner for Mr. Pritikin at the Kaneohe Yacht Club in Kaneohe, Hawaii. More than 225 people, many of whom were my patients, made McDougall-style meals. He said he loved the food. After dinner we walked together to his car to say good-bye. Mary gave him approximately a hundred of her recipes. At that time the food served at the Pritikin Center in Santa Monica, California, had a reputation for being unimaginative and, to Pritikin's continued frustration, tasteless. In his next book, *The Pritikin Promise* (1983), he incorporated some of Mary's recipes into his program. I believe that it was no coincidence that the food served at the Pritikin Center improved greatly afterward.

My First Residential Program: St. Helena Hospital

In 1986, the Seventh-Day Adventist St. Helena Hospital in Napa Valley, California, invited me to run the McDougall Program, a lifestyle residential program designed to improve health, help people lose excess body weight, and get people off unnecessary medications. My protocol aligned perfectly with the Seventh-Day Adventists' advocacy of a vegetarian diet and a healthy lifestyle for its religious congregants. (I am not an Adventist.) The St. Helena Hospital was also considered one of the best heart-surgery centers in the country. Even then it seemed odd to me that they would invite a doctor who is against most heart surgeries to work at a hospital that makes 80 percent of its income from heart disease.

Now that I was working at a nationally respected hospital, I figured I might be able to convince health insurers to cover the cost of my program for patients. I approached several well-known companies, arguing that our program could treat heart patients at a fraction of the cost of bypass surgery ($4,000 vs. $80,000). No matter how hard I tried to convince them, however, I couldn't get anyone to bite. A representative from one large insurer told me that his company was not interested in my approach because it required the cooperation of the patient, and all the bypass surgeon had to do to relieve chest pain was to get the patient to willingly lie down on the operating room table. To my surprise, doctors and health providers had little faith in patients' judgment and willpower. "But some patients will change their diet, and they deserve this alternative," I countered. That's when I finally got the real reason health insurance providers refused my offer.

"McDougall," one frustrated insurer told me, "you just don't get it. As an insurance company, we take a piece of the pie, and the bigger the pie, the more we get."

During my sixteen years at St. Helena, I was able to talk to some of the best heart surgeons and cardiologists in the country—some of whom I still consider my friends. On several occasions, I offered to refer my patients to them for a second opinion, and I expected them to return the favor. I got no takers. Although a kind radiologist confided, "We know your diet works. We see the repeat angiograms of their heart arteries showing reversal." Other doctors saw no need to have their patients receive instruction on healthier eating (from me or anyone else).

I have fond memories of those years working at the hospital. On many occasions, I cared for the physicians there as well as their spouses and children. And the talented and caring professional staff helped thousands of people while I was there. But, within this setting, the number of those in my program never seemed to grow as I wanted. Maybe people saw a contradiction between health (my program) and medical treatment (the hospital), as if the two fields were mutually exclusive. Even though I was becoming a national figure, appearing at that time on most of the top TV and radio shows around the country to promote my best-selling books, the number of our participants was far lower than it should have been.

In 2002, Roy Swank, the inventor of the Swank Diet, a low-saturated-fat dietary treatment for multiple sclerosis, invited me to incorporate his patient population into my live-in program, which would have doubled or tripled the number of patients attending my clinic at St. Helena Hospital. Because this was a win-win opportunity for everyone, I expected an enthusiastic response from the hospital administration.

After lengthy discussions, however, hospital administrators told me that they did not want to be associated with MS patients. At first I thought they were afraid of the stigma attached to this debilitating disease. But I eventually realized the real reason was that treating MS patients didn't generate significant profits. I explained that our primary purpose as a hospital was to treat the sick, and because of the Adventist orientation we were called to treat our patients with a vegetarian diet therapy—there was no greater match between mission and practice. But the administrators were steadfast. Five days later, when it was time to renew my contract, I submitted it with "Void" written over the front page.

Later I was told they had assumed I would never leave their hospital setting, because they wrongly believed I couldn't run the McDougall Program without their organization.

The McDougall Program

The truth was, I had run the McDougall Program many times without the hospital. Between 1999 and 2001, for instance, I ran my program near Minneapolis for the medical insurance company Blue Cross Blue Shield. During this three-year period, with three different employee groups within the company, I was able to show the same remarkable health benefits we were getting at St. Helena Hospital: weight loss; reduction in cholesterol, blood pressure, and blood sugars; and relief from indigestion, constipation, and arthritis, among other short- and long-term benefits. What's more, I was also able to document a 44 percent reduction in health-care costs for each of the three groups based on the insurance company's own claims data.

I had had a similar experience in Lakeland, Florida, where I cared for some of the employees of Publix Supermarkets. Both of these remote programs were run out of local hotels. Within seventy-two hours, I can set up a ten-day McDougall Program anywhere. The only thing the program requires are sensible people looking to regain their lost health and appearance.

In May of 2002 I launched the first McDougall Program at the Flamingo Resort in Santa Rosa, California. The number of our participants doubled in no time. The food now tastes as if Mary made it at home. Like many things in life, we have asked ourselves why we waited so long to take over complete control of our program. We have gone on to accomplish so much and have built a devoted following in the process.

Our nonprofit foundation (501c3) raises money to complete research projects, such as the 2013 study with OHSU on the dietary treatment of multiple sclerosis,[6] and the results of 1,615 people who attended our ten-day McDougall residential program, which we published in the October 2014 issue of *Nutrition Journal*.[7] Our foundation also pays for medical students and training residents to take a monthlong learning experience with us at our residential program. The website www.drmcdougall.com receives half a million hits a month. We have more than 115,000 "likes" on Facebook. Dr. McDougall's Right Foods (a packaged meal system in paper cups) are sold in over 6,000 stores nationwide. Our free newsletter goes out to more than 64,000 people monthly. Thousands of people tune in to our weekly free webinars. And we make new friends every month at our ten-day medical live-in programs, three-day programs, Advanced Study Weekends, and Travel Adventure trips. It sure seems like we're on the right track.

3

The Healthiest Diet Versus Fad Diets

When I first looked closely at my patients on the Hamakua Sugar Plantation on the Big Island of Hawaii, I realized they had a lot in common. Most of them, regardless of age, worked physically demanding jobs, and they observed many of the same customs. The single difference between the older and younger generations was their diet.

The older patients followed the traditional diet of their ancestors. Their regimens were based primarily on plant foods, most prominently grains (like rice), fresh vegetables, beans, and fruits. The younger generation, meanwhile, lived on a modern diet based heavily on animal foods and vegetable oils. They also ate significant amounts of processed and refined foods loaded with fat, sugar, salt, and artificial ingredients. I knew that the food was the culprit and not genetics, because if genes were the cause of disease, all generations—young and old alike—would have exhibited the same common chronic illnesses. But that wasn't the case. Only the younger generation, the men, women, and children who subsisted on the modern Western diet, was deteriorating in rapid fashion.

Given the right diet and lifestyle, the body will recover. When we remove the poisons from our lives and replace them with health-promoting foods, the ones featured in the Healthiest Diet on the Planet, the body can and will begin to heal itself—even from illnesses often widely deemed "incurable."

And yet, instead of following my simple and delicious protocol—a protocol that continues to help hundreds of thousands, if not millions, of people a year—people continue to get caught up in the newest fad diets, which sets them back even more in their quest for lifelong health and vibrant longevity. So let's settle this once and for all. Let's compare the Healthiest Diet on the Planet to three of today's most popular and touted diets, all of which—for one reason or another—feature meat as their centerpiece: the Wheat Belly Diet, the Grain Brain Diet, and the Paleo Diet.

The Wheat Belly and Grain Brain Diets

Robert Atkins, M.D., the man behind the famous Atkins Diet, was upfront with his recommendations. In his original version in the 1970s, he wanted people to eat a diet almost exclusively made up of meat, poultry, cheese, butter, fish, eggs, and vegetable oils, with no carbohydrates (plant foods).[1] The first Atkins Diet book was published in 1972; since then well-informed people have come to understand, through their own research and personal experiences, that eating a high-fat, low-carbohydrate, animal-based diet is wrong. Following this eating pattern, they have learned, causes our epidemic diseases, including obesity, type 2 diabetes, coronary heart disease, and common cancers (breast, prostate, and colon). They also learn, if they dig just a little bit deeper, that the livestock industry is

Low-Carbohydrate Diets Increase the Risk of Death and Disease

The article "Low-Carbohydrate Diets and All-Cause and Cause-Specific Mortality," published in the *Annals of Internal Medicine* (2010), concludes: A low-carbohydrate diet based on animal sources was associated with higher all-cause mortality.[2]

"Low-Carbohydrate, High-Protein Diet and Incidence of Cardiovascular Diseases in Swedish Women: Prospective Cohort Study," in the *British Medical Journal* (2012), warns: "Low-carbohydrate, high-protein diets, used on a regular basis . . . are associated with increased risk of cardiovascular disease."[3]

The highly respected *PLOS One* journal, in the article "Low-Carbohydrate Diets and All-Cause Mortality: A Systematic Review and Meta-Analysis of Observational Studies" (2013), reports: "Low-carbohydrate diets were associated with a significantly higher risk of all-cause mortality."[4]

"Low-Carbohydrate Diet from Plant or Animal Sources and Mortality Among Myocardial Infarction (MI) Survivors," in the *Journal of the American Heart Association* (2014), maintains: "Greater adherence to an LCD (low-carbohydrate diet) high in animal sources of fat and protein was associated with higher all-cause and cardiovascular mortality post-MI."[5]

at the root of climate change, the decline of our ecosystems, and the loss of species worldwide. Many people are also now wrestling with their conscience as they deal with the moral issues of factory farming, where animals are being cruelly treated and killed unnecessarily for food, and the depletion of our oceans: 90 percent of the large fish have been lost since my childhood in the 1950s.

But the Atkins Diet, which so many people have since rightly dismissed, still lives on, though it has since taken different forms. Dr. Atkins was direct in his dietary advice, but Dr. William Davis, author of *Wheat Belly: Lose the Wheat, Lose the Weight, and Find Your Path Back to Health,* and Dr. David Perlmutter, author of *Grain Brain: The Surprising Truth about Wheat, Carbs, and Sugar—Your Brain's Silent Killers,* take a backdoor approach to the Atkins high-fat, low-carbohydrate way of eating.[6] As the titles of these best-selling books suggest, wheat causes a big belly, while grains damage the brain. Within their respective pages, Dr. Davis and Dr. Perlmutter argue that starchy foods, most notably wheat, rice, corn, and potatoes—the traditional foods consumed by billions of people throughout human history—are unhealthy and should be eaten only sparingly, if not avoided altogether.

If you believe Dr. Davis and Dr. Perlmutter, then what is left to eat in order to meet your energy requirements? That's right: animal-derived foods and vegetable oils, the primary components of the original Atkins Diet. A few fruits and nonstarchy vegetables (broccoli, Brussels sprouts, celery, kale, lettuce, parsley, peppers, and zucchini and other colorful vegetables) are commonly added to these newer low-carbohydrate diets in an effort to partially compensate for obvious nutritional deficiencies found in the original Atkins Diet (which lacks dietary fiber, vitamin C, essential carbohydrates, and

Animal Foods, Not Plant Foods, Cause Inflammation

The *European Journal of Nutrition* published the article "Consumption of Red Meat and Whole-Grain Bread in Relation to Biomarkers of Obesity, Inflammation, Glucose Metabolism, and Oxidative Stress" (2013). The results of this study suggest that high consumption of whole-grain bread is related to lower levels of inflammatory markers that are associated with worse health.[7]

"Dietary Pattern Analysis and Biomarkers of Low-Grade Inflammation: A Systematic Literature Review" appeared in *Nutrition Reviews* (2013). A major conclusion: patterns identified by reduced rank regression as being statistically and significantly associated with biomarkers of inflammation were almost all meat-based or due to "Western" eating patterns.[8]

The *American Journal of Clinical Nutrition* published the article "Associations between Red Meat Intake and Biomarkers of Inflammation and Glucose Metabolism in Women" (2014). It concludes that greater red meat intake is associated with unfavorable plasma concentrations of inflammatory and glucose metabolic biomarkers in diabetes-free women.[9]

According to "The Protein Type within a Hypocaloric Diet Affects Obesity-Related Inflammation: The RESMENA Project," published in the journal *Nutrition* (2014), total protein intake was positively associated with inflammation as well as with animal protein.[10]

The *British Journal of Nutrition* published the article "Non-Soya Legume-Based Therapeutic Lifestyle Change (TLC) Diet Reduces Inflammatory Status in Diabetic Patients: A Randomised Cross-Over Clinical Trial" (2015). Its conclusion: the replacement of two servings of red meat by nonsoya legumes in the isoenergetic TLC diet for a period of three days per week reduced the plasma concentrations of inflammatory markers among overweight diabetic patients, independent of weight change.[11]

A *Journal of the National Academy of Sciences USA* article entitled "A Red Meat-Derived Glycan Promotes Inflammation and Cancer Progression" (2015) maintains that similar mechanisms may contribute to the association of red meat consumption with other diseases, such as atherosclerosis and type 2 diabetes, which are also exacerbated by inflammation.[12]

thousands of other phytochemicals). Starches (beans, corn, potatoes, and rice) are the primary source of carbohydrates; thus "low-carbohydrate" is in practical terms synonymous with meat, poultry, cheese, butter, fish, eggs, and vegetable oils.

In order for the authors of these two books to pull off the monumental task of luring otherwise intelligent people back into inherently dangerous diet plans, they have had to: (1) ignore the bulk of the science, (2) exaggerate the truth, and (3) make false associations.

Ignoring the Science

Although low-carbohydrate diets can cause weight loss, weight loss should not be the primary goal of individuals, medical doctors, dietitians, insurance companies, or governments. The goal is to

Grains (Including Wheat) Do Not Increase Inflammation

The article "Whole Grains Are Associated with Serum Concentrations of High Sensitivity C-reactive Protein among Premenopausal Women," published in the *Journal of Nutrition* (2010), concludes that women who consumed more than one serving of whole grains a day had a lower probability of having moderate or elevated markers of inflammation compared with nonconsumers.[13]

"Effect of Whole Grains on Markers of Subclinical Inflammation," published in *Nutrition Reviews* (2012), reveals that epidemiological studies provide reasonable support for an association between diets high in whole grains and lower concentrations of markers of inflammation.[14]

Nutrition Journal published the article "The Potential Role of Phytochemicals in Whole-Grain Cereals for the Prevention of Type-2 Diabetes" (2013). Its conclusions were that diets high in whole grains are associated with a 20–30 percent reduction in the risk of developing type 2 diabetes, and biomarkers of systemic inflammation tend to be reduced in people consuming high intakes of whole grains.[15]

The *Journal of Medicinal Food* published a review article on five grains, "Bioactives in Commonly Consumed Cereal Grains: Implications for Oxidative Stress and Inflammation" (2015). It states: "We suggest that grains, which are a great source of antioxidants, have potential in the prevention of oxidative stress and inflammation-related chronic diseases."[16]

Whole grains are consistently found to be healthy. A recent review of forty-five prospective cohort studies and twenty-one randomized-controlled trials compared people who rarely or never consume whole grains with those reporting an average consumption of three to five servings per day. Examples of whole grains included wheat, oats, brown rice, rye, barley, and bulgur. Using comprehensive meta-analysis, the review found that those consuming the grains had a 26 percent reduction in the risk of type 2 diabetes and a 21 percent reduction in the risk of heart disease. Furthermore, there is an inverse relationship between whole-grain intake and weight gain.[17]

live long and stay healthy. Major scientific reviews show that low-carbohydrate diets increase the risk of sickness and death (see box on page 52).

Note that there are no similar scientific reviews condemning high-carbohydrate diets such as the Healthiest Diet on the Planet. This is because the diet I recommend for you is the natural way humans eat and thus prevents diseases caused by "food poisoning" from eating animal foods and vegetable oils. Most important, once these unhealthy foods are avoided, the body heals.

Exaggerating the Truth about Inflammation

Promoters of low-carbohydrate diets claim dietary carbohydrates are packed with inflammatory ingredients and that inflammation is at the heart of virtually every disorder and disease. The evidence linking carbohydrates to inflammation is convoluted, theoretical, and largely limited to celiac disease, an uncommon condition that prevents the small intestine from effectively absorbing necessary nutrients, leading to diarrhea, abdominal pain, flatulence, weakness, and weight loss.[18]

Inflammation is the consequence of injury, such as a cut, burn, or infection. The pain, redness, swelling, and heat that follow are natural, necessary processes for healing. These symptoms and signs of inflammation resolve after the single event. However, with repetitive injury, inflammation can become long-standing, which is referred to as "chronic inflammation." One common example of chronic inflammation is bronchitis that results from inhaling cigarette smoke twenty times a day. If you stop smoking, the repeated injury stops, then the inflammation stops, and the lungs start to heal immediately, although scar tissue and other residuals of the damage can remain.

When it comes to dietary-caused inflammation, scientific research solidly and consistently blames meat, poultry, dairy, and eggs as the sources of the repeated injury and the resulting chronic inflammation (see boxes on pages 54 and 55). The diseases that follow include coronary heart disease, type 2 diabetes, cancer, and inflammatory arthritis. Fortunately, once the source of injury is stopped, the inflammation resolves, and healing occurs. The research does not support the theory that carbohydrates from wheat, other grains, or starchy vegetables lead to chronic inflammation (see boxes on pages 56 and 57). No debate here.

Making False Associations
Based on Celiac Disease

Low-carb diet proponents often use celiac disease to demonize all carbohydrates for all people. The main takeaway that readers will get from *Wheat Belly* is that wheat is the major cause of obesity, heart disease, diabetes, and almost all other major and minor health problems. Although wheat can be very troublesome for a small percentage of the population, celiac disease affects fewer than one in one hundred people following the Western diet.[19] These people must avoid gluten, which is found in high concentrations in wheat, barley, and rye. However, to put this real concern into a global historical perspective, consider the importance of these three grains: they have served to fuel the development of civilizations throughout human history and still serve as a major source of calories, protein, vitamins, and minerals for billions of people. People without celiac disease or the very few other conditions that warrant elimination of these three specific grains will find them an excellent and tasty source of nutrition.

Patients with celiac disease are usually suffering from malnourishment because of the problems created by damage to their intestines from gluten. Following removal of wheat, barley, and rye, the gastrointestinal tract usually heals, and only then are calories and other nutrients efficiently assimilated so that weight can be gained. Weight gain is the desired and expected outcome for underweight people with celiac disease.

Some people with documented celiac disease, however, are overweight and even obese before starting a gluten-free diet. You might expect that the dietary restrictions imposed by a strict gluten-free protocol alone would cause weight loss for them. Unfortunately, weight gain is a common occurrence in overweight and obese adults and children with celiac disease who go on gluten-free diets.[20] A 2012 study of 1,018 patients with biopsy-confirmed celiac disease found significant weight gain in 22 percent of patients after starting their new gluten-free diet.[21] To reiterate this point, a 2011 article in the *Journal of the American Dietetic Association* states, "At this time there is no scientific evidence supporting the alleged benefit that a gluten-free diet will promote weight loss."[22]

The primary reason for unwanted weight gain found in people buying gluten-free products is that these imitations often contain as much or more calories, fat, and sugar and fewer important nutrients, such as dietary fiber, complex carbohydrates, vitamins, and minerals, than the original gluten-containing foods (see box on page 61). Even the casual observer can see the folly in eating gluten-free cakes, cookies, and pies and expecting weight loss and better health. A trip through your local health-food store or supermarket reveals rows of desserts in which the wheat has been replaced with another grain (flour), and fats, vegetable oils, simple sugars, dairy products, and eggs are abundant on the ingredient lists. Estimates as high as 15–25 percent are given for the number of consumers in the United States who want gluten-free food.[23]

Although I applaud Dr. Davis for bringing problems with wheat to greater public awareness for the very few who would benefit, I consider this fad a serious diversion away from what I believe to be the real solution to obesity and common diseases: a starch-based diet. Traditionally my kind of high-carbohydrate eating has been the diet of people throughout recorded human history, and a large share of these populations, ancient and modern, have relied on generous amounts of wheat, barley, and/or rye for survival.

While exaggerating the benefits of a wheat-free diet, Dr. Davis makes clear his alliance with the low-carb movement made popular by Dr. Atkins. Dr. Davis recommends people eat unlimited amounts

Percent of Calories from Fat in Popular Gluten-Free Foods

Falafel..71 percent

Chocolate Chip Cookies ....50 percent

Chocolate Cake.. 38 percent

Brownies... 38 percent

Cupcakes .... 37 percent

Cheese Pizza.. 36 percent

These foods also can contain fattening and health-harming saturated fats, isolated vegetable oils, simple sugars, refined flours, nuts, soy products, dairy products, and eggs.

of eggs, full-fat cheese, other dairy products, meat, fish, chicken, and vegetable (olive) oils.[24] My opposite conclusion is that these same rich foods, once reserved for the tables of opulent kings and queens, are actually the cause of the current epidemics of obesity and common illnesses in the developed world.

When an expert dietitian knowledgeable about proper food choices for a healthy gluten-free diet devoid of cakes, cookies, and pies is involved in patient care, then weight loss is accomplished. In one study, overweight and obese patients were advised to choose a high-quality gluten-free diet with naturally gluten-free foods (fruits and vegetables) and non-gluten-containing grains (quinoa and buckwheat). These properly counseled patients consistently lost excess weight.[25] There is unfortunately a paucity of dietitians and medical doctors available for the proper management of celiac disease or any of the epidemic diseases caused by the rich Western diet.

The fad to "go gluten-free," however, can indirectly harm many celiac patients. If you are one of the few people with celiac disease, then avoiding gluten is crucial to your health. You cannot cheat! But with the popularity of going gluten-free for unsubstantiated reasons, the importance of this dietary restriction for the truly needy has been diminished. One way this happens is when waiters at restaurants become used to customers asking for "gluten-free" dishes and then failing to object when a few whole wheat bread crumbs appear

McDougall Foods Acceptable for Those with Celiac Disease

GRAINS:

Amaranth	Quinoa
Buckwheat (or kasha)	Rice
Corn	Sorghum
Job's tears	Teff
Millet	Wild rice
Oats (certified gluten-free)	

OTHER FOODS:

All root vegetables, like potatoes, yams, sweet potatoes, and cassava root (tapioca)

All legumes, more specifically, beans (including soybeans and chickpeas), peas, and lentils

All green and yellow vegetables

All fruits

on top of their potato soup. Since wheat, barley, and rye did not cause any apparent distress in the previous ninety-nine customers, the waiters and chefs think, "It can't be all that important." But for that single celiac customer, it is.

If you suspect that you have celiac disease, then get tested by your physician. Avoidance of foods with gluten is a lifelong restriction. If you are unsure about your diagnosis, but still suspect a gluten sensitivity, then go on a starch-based diet with no wheat, barley, or rye. For example, you can base your diet on corn, rice, sweet potatoes, potatoes, and/or beans, adding some fruits and green and yellow vegetables. The connection between gluten and celiac disease is so close that the diagnosis can often be made when the patient experiences dramatic improvement of symptoms upon following a gluten-free diet (see box on page 62). Confirmation of your diagnosis can be made by carefully adding back any suspected foods.

If you, like two-thirds of adults in the United States, are sick and overweight and if you, like the vast majority, do not have celiac disease, a wheat allergy, or a wheat sensitivity, then I strongly recommend that you include wheat, barley, and rye in your diet, because these good starches are known to cause desirable weight loss and confer medical benefits.

Making False Associations Between Diabetes and Carbohydrates

The main takeaway that readers will get from *Grain Brain* is that grains and other starchy foods are the cause of type 2 diabetes, Alzheimer's disease, obesity, and most of the other chronic health problems suffered in the Western world.[26] The truth is that people with type 2 diabetes are ill with many disorders of the body and brain, but grains and other starchy vegetables do not cause type 2 diabetes. The Western diet, loaded with meat, fat, and empty calories, makes people overweight and then causes them to go on to develop type 2 diabetes. The same diet, independently, causes heart disease, common cancers, and brain disorders, including strokes and Alzheimer's disease. Rice and other starches actually prevent, and often times cure, common chronic diseases suffered by Americans and others worldwide.

Type 2 diabetes is cured by a starch-based, high-carbohydrate diet.[27] To take this point to the extreme, Dr. Kempner's Rice Diet, which consists of white rice, fruit, fruit juice, and table sugar—more than 90 percent of the calories are from carbohydrates—has been shown to cause profound weight loss in the severely obese, cure type 2 diabetes, and reverse heart disease.[28] High-carbohydrate diets are inherently low in fat. Dietary fat, freely recommended in the *Wheat Belly* and *Grain Brain* programs, actually increases blood-sugar levels and causes people with type 1 diabetes to require more insulin.[29]

Regardless of the effects on blood sugar, the underlying animal-based, low-grain, low-starch diet consisting of those very foods recommended in *Wheat Belly* and *Grain Brain* is the major reason people with type 2 diabetes are so sick with heart and other diseases.[30]

The common denominator: *it's the food!*

Looking Beyond the Smoke and Mirrors

The truth is that the rich Western diet makes people fat and sick. Steering people away from the few healthy components of our diet (grains and other starchy vegetables) and toward the most unhealthy foods (meat, poultry, dairy, fish, eggs, and vegetable oils) makes matters worse. People are desperate for a solution to their weight and health problems, and many of them are easily deceived. People love to hear good news about their bad habits—they love to be told that prime rib and cheddar cheese are good for them. But the bottom line is that the rising popularity of low-carbohydrate diets and books like *Wheat Belly* and *Grain Brain* enhance the profits of the meat, poultry, dairy, fish, egg, and vegetable oil industries. Secondarily, hospitals, health-care professionals, and pharmaceutical and device companies rake in great profits from all this illness caused by eating animal-derived foods and vegetable oils.

Although these industries spend billions of dollars advertising "their science" and influencing national nutrition and health policies, the truth is simple and easy to understand: all large, successfully trim healthy populations of people throughout human history have obtained the bulk of their calories from grains and other starchy vegetables. Consumption of meats along with other rich foods in any significant quantity has been the prerogative of fat and sick kings, queens, and aristocrats—until recently. To regain our lost health and save Planet Earth, the smoke and mirrors behind popular diet books must be exposed.

The Paleo Diet

The Paleo Diet (also referred to as the Paleolithic Diet, the Paleodiet, the Caveman Diet, the Stone Age Diet, and the Hunter-Gatherer Diet) is a widely popular approach to weight loss, improved health, and longevity. The diet consists mainly of meat, poultry, shellfish,

Recent Research Reveals Ancient Populations Were Starch Eaters

Research published in the journal *Nature* reports that almost the entire diet of our very early human ancestors, dating to two million years ago, consisted of leaves, fruits, wood, and bark—a diet similar to that of modern-day chimpanzees.[31]

According to research presented in a 2009 issue of *Science*, people living in what is now Mozambique, along the eastern coast of Africa, may have followed a diet based on the cereal grass sorghum as early as 105,000 years ago.[32]

Research presented in a 2011 issue of *Proceedings of the National Academy of Sciences* shows that even Neanderthals ate a variety of plant foods; starch grains have been found on their skeletal teeth everywhere from the warm eastern Mediterranean to chilly northwestern Europe.[33] It appears they even cooked and otherwise prepared plant foods to make them more digestible—44,000 years ago.

A 2010 issue of the *Proceedings of the National Academy of Sciences* reported that starch grains from wild plants were identified on grinding tools at archaeological sites dating back to the Paleolithic period in Italy, Russia, and the Czech Republic.[34] These findings suggest that processing vegetables and starches, possibly grinding them into flour, was a widespread practice in Europe as far back as 30,000 years ago or even earlier.

In 2013 the *National Academy of Sciences USA* published an article, "Paleolithic Human Exploitation of Plant Foods during the Last Glacial Maximum in North China," showing that, 23,000 to 19,500 calendar years before the present, people depended heavily on plant foods, especially beans and tubers (yams) for food.[35]

A 2015 issue of the *Proceedings of the National Academy of Sciences USA* contained an article, "Multistep Food Plant Processing at Grotta Paglicci (Southern Italy) Around 32,600 Cal B.P." It found: "The study clearly indicates that the exploitation of plant resources was very important for hunter-gatherer populations, to the point that the Early Gravettian inhabitants of Paglicci were able to process food plants and already possessed a wealth of knowledge that was to become widespread after the dawn of agriculture."[36]

fish, and eggs; nonstarchy orange, green, and yellow vegetables; and fruits and nuts.[37] This approach forbids starches, including all grains, legumes, and potatoes. To its credit it also excludes dairy products and refined sugars. Salt and processed oils are also excluded, with the exception of olive oil.

This nutritional plan is based on the presumption that our ancestors, living during the Paleolithic era—between 2.5 million and 10,000 years ago—were nourished primarily by animal foods. According to the basic theory behind Paleo, as a result of more than two million years of evolution, we are now genetically adapted to eat what the hunter-gatherers ate—mostly animal foods.

The Paleo Diet: Lose Weight and Get Healthy by Eating the Foods You Were Designed to Eat (revised 2011) is the bible for followers of this approach. Written by Loren Cordain, Ph.D., a professor in the Department of Health and Exercise Science at Colorado State University, the Paleo Diet is said to be "the one and only diet that ideally fits our genetic makeup."[38] The author claims that every human being on earth ate this way for the past 2.5 million years, until the dawn of the Agricultural Revolution (10,000 years ago), when grains, legumes, and potatoes were introduced worldwide. According to Dr. Cordain, "There wasn't a single person who did *not* follow the Paleo Diet." Paleo "experts" teach that human health and longevity plummeted with the development of agriculture. By no coincidence, the Agricultural Revolution marks the dawn of civilization. "Civilization" encompasses our advanced state of intellectual, cultural, and material development, marked by progress in the arts, music, sciences, languages, writing, computers, transportation, and politics.

Teachers of Paleo nutrition claim our ancient ancestors were hunter-gatherers with an emphasis on hunting, regardless of what the bulk of current scientific research reports. They base their hypothesis largely upon a flawed review of contemporary hunter-gatherers.[39]

Primates, including humans, have practiced hunting and gathering for millions of years. I know of no large populations of primates who have been strict vegans. However, plants have, with very few exceptions, provided the bulk of the calories for almost all primates. This truth has been unpopular in part because of a well-recognized human trait: sexism. Grandparents, women, and children did the gathering, while men hunted. Glory always goes to the (men) hunters.

When asked about the commonly held idea that ancient people were primarily meat eaters, the highly respected anthropologist Nathaniel Dominy, Ph.D., from Dartmouth College, responded, "That's a myth. Hunter-gatherers, the majority of their calories come from plant foods. . . . Meat is just too unpredictable." After studying the bones, teeth, and genetics of primates for his entire career as a biological anthropologist, Dr. Dominy states, "Humans might be more appropriately described as 'starchivores.'"[40]

Paleo Diet proponents spare no effort to ignore and distort science.[41] The general public is at their mercy until they look at recent publications from the major scientific journals (see box on pages 66 and 67).

The September 2015 issue of the *Quarterly Review of Biology* contained a very thorough review of the importance of dietary carbohydrate in human evolution (a must-read article and free over the Internet; search: "The Importance of Dietary Carbohydrate in Human Evolution"). Even the article's abstract confirms the science behind the Healthiest Diet on the Planet and refutes popular diet books that claim the opposite:

> We propose that plant foods containing high quantities
> of starch were essential for the evolution of the human
> phenotype during the Pleistocene (from 2.6 million to 12,000
> years ago). Although previous studies have highlighted a
> stone tool–mediated shift from primarily plant-based to
> primarily meat-based diets as critical in the development of
> the brain and other human traits, we argue that digestible
> carbohydrates were also necessary to accommodate
> the increased metabolic demands of a growing brain.
> Furthermore, we acknowledge the adaptive role cooking
> played in improving the digestibility and palatability of key
> carbohydrates. We provide evidence that cooked starch,
> a source of preformed glucose, greatly increased energy
> availability to human tissues with high glucose demands,

such as the brain, red blood cells, and the developing fetus. We also highlight the auxiliary role [that] copy number variation in the salivary amylase genes may have played in increasing the importance of starch in human evolution following the origins of cooking.[42]

This paragraph can be a little hard to digest, but it is a landmark review for those who truly are interested in showing the fallacies behind the thinking of people promoting the avoidance of starches as a way to regain their lost health.

A Repulsive Diet

More than half (55 percent) of a Paleo dieter's food comes from lean meats, organ meats, fish, and seafood. "For most of us," Dr. Cordain writes, "the thought of eating organs is not only repulsive, but is also not practical, as we simply do not have access to wild game."[43] In addition to the usual beef, veal, pork, chicken, and fish, a Paleo follower is encouraged to eat alligator, bear, kangaroo, deer, rattlesnake, and wild boar. Mail-order suppliers for these wild animals are provided in his book. Bone marrow and brains of animals were both favorites of precivilization hunter-gatherers. For most of us (including the Paleo dieters), the thought of eating bone marrow and brains is repulsive.

In addition, no mention is made by Paleo experts about the frequent and habitual practices of nutritional cannibalism by hunter-gatherer societies.[44] (Nutritional cannibalism refers to the consumption of human flesh for its taste or nutritional value.)

Archaeologists have found bones of our ancestors from a million years ago with defleshing marks and evidence of bone smashing to get at the marrow inside; there are signs that the brains of victims were also eaten (and children were not off the menu). And we are supposed to eat the favorite meats of our uncivilized, pre–Agricultural Revolution hunter-gatherer ancestors?

A Nutritional Nightmare

By nature, the Paleo Diet is based on artery-clogging saturated fats and cholesterol and bone-damaging, acidic proteins from animal foods. Respected researchers find that modern-day hunter-gatherer populations who base their diets on meat, such as the Inuits (Eskimos), suffer from heart disease and other forms of atherosclerosis.[45] Also epidemic among meat- and fish-consuming hunter-gatherers, specifically the Inuits, is osteoporosis.[46] Meanwhile, hunter-gatherers who base their diets on plant foods (starches) are free of these diseases.[47]

Impending Ecological Disaster

The 2006 report *Livestock's Long Shadow: Environmental Issues and Options,* by the Food and Agriculture Organization of the United Nations, concludes: "Livestock have a substantial impact on the world's water, land and biodiversity resources and contribute significantly to climate change. Animal agriculture produces 18 percent of the world's greenhouse gas emissions (CO_2 equivalents), compared with 13.5 percent from all forms of transportation combined."[48]

This report is a conservative estimate of the destruction caused by the very foods that *Wheat Belly, Grain Brain,* and *The Paleo Diet* recommend in abundance. Calculations by the World Watch Institute find that over 51 percent of the global-warming gases are the result of raising animals for people to eat.[49] In March 2016, an article in the *Proceedings of the National Academy of Sciences* concluded that the transition toward a plant-based diet could reduce global mortality by as much as 10 percent and food-related greenhouse-gas emissions by as much as 70 percent and result in economic benefits reaching as high as $31 trillion by 2050.[50] Every person whom Paleo gurus convince to follow an animal food–based diet brings us one step closer to the end of the world as we know it.

Civilization Would Not Have Evolved

According to Dr. Cordain, "The Agricultural Revolution changed the world and allowed civilizations—cities, culture, technological and medical achievements, and scientific knowledge—to develop."[51] In other words, if people had remained on a diet of mostly animal foods (assuming this was the diet of our ancestors), we would still be living in the Stone Age. Fortunately, the Agricultural Revolution, with the efficient production of grains, legumes, and potatoes—the very foods recommended by the Healthiest Diet on the Planet—allowed us to become civilized.

Dr. Cordain finishes the 2011 revision of his national best-selling book *The Paleo Diet* by warning, "Without them (starches, like wheat, rice, corn, and potatoes), the world could probably support one-tenth or less of our present population."[52] Choose ten close friends and family members. Which nine should die so that the Paleo people can have their way?

The Healthiest Diet on the Planet is the better way. In the following pages, I will share a visual guide that makes it very clear what we should eat and what we should avoid.

Red Light, Green Light

Dr. McDougall's Guide to What We Should and Shouldn't Eat

Change begins with opening our eyes so we can see. This happened for me as a senior medical student at a noontime hospital conference in 1971, when I heard Dr. Denis Burkitt describe his experiences with the people of Uganda, who had none of the common Western diseases because they lived on a starch-based diet. It took me another six years, following my experiences as a sugar-plantation doctor and becoming a board-certified internist, before I clearly understood that this simple truth could prevent, and usually cure, more than 80 percent of the health problems Americans suffer from, including obesity, type 2 diabetes, heart disease, common cancers, and intestinal disorders.

Since then I have tried to help others see this truth through the millions of words in my best-selling books and monthly newsletters, on my popular website, and delivered at more than a thousand live lectures. Two of my favorite quotes are: "The truth is simple and easy to understand" and "Pictures are worth a thousand words." It has taken me nearly forty years to apply this common knowledge to my life's work.

While on a McDougall Travel Adventure trip to Costa Rica in June 2014, I developed and presented for the first time to 140 fellow travelers my slide presentation, *Dr. McDougall's Color Picture Book: "Food Poisoning" and How to Cure It by Eating Beans, Corn, Pasta, Potatoes, Rice, Etc.* Before publishing this lecture in my June 2014 *McDougall Newsletter,* I sat down with my three oldest grandsons, ages six, eight, and ten, and showed them my picture book. (I have seven grandchildren.) I asked them, "Do you know what the three traffic lights, red, yellow, and green, mean?" (I have placed these three colors with the pictures that follow.)

"Yes, Grandpa. They mean stop, caution, and go."

I then went over the pictures, saying a few brief words about each page. "Do you understand what to eat, what not to eat, and why?"

"Yes, Grandpa," each one responded. (They liked the picture about constipation best.)

Since then I have presented this talk more than a hundred times to lay and professional audiences. The response has been overwhelmingly positive. People very much appreciate the straightforward delivery of this lifesaving information; some even call it "genius" in its simplicity. This simple-to-understand message consists of almost seventy pictures with a few words, is able to be viewed in less than fifteen minutes, and has been translated into more than twenty-three languages on my website, www.drmcdougall.com. However, this is the first time my *Color Picture Book* has been available in book form for the general public. My guess is that it has already changed hundreds of thousands of lives. With the readership expected thanks to HarperOne, millions of lives will be dramatically turned around, and this simple little book will become a crucial addition to everyone's efforts to save Planet Earth.

The livestock industry accounts for a majority of global damage, and by changing the food we eat, this source of damage could be halted immediately. If all eyes were opened, then the world's population could switch from obtaining their calories from animal foods to obtaining them from starches overnight—giving us the breathing room we need to solve energy and transportation problems before we become extinct. Please share the Healthiest Diet on the Planet with family, friends, and people you meet on the street. Every person counts.

Red Light, Green Light

Dr. McDougall's Guide to What We Should and Shouldn't Eat

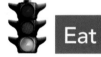 **Don't Eat**

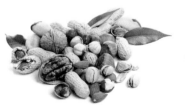 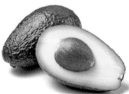 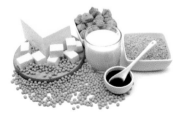

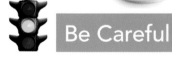 **Eat**

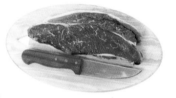 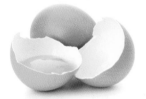 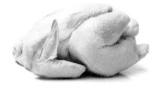

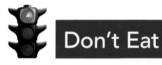 **Be Careful**

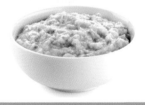 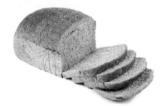 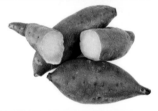

> Forget about being reasonable, sensible, prudent, or moderate. You can't!

You Must Fix the Food

- Moderation does not work for changing life-destroying habits.

- Cigarette smokers never quit by cutting down.

- Alcoholics do not sober up by switching to beer or wine.

- You must treat "food poisoning" with the same good or evil, right or wrong, go or stop, green or red attitude as you would use to treat drug addiction.

Just say NO to the foods that are poisoning you and your family.

The truth is simple and easy to understand:

- The Healthiest Diet on the Planet
  is based on starches with vegetables and fruits.

- The Healthiest Diet on the Planet
  does not contain any animal foods or vegetable oils.

- The Healthiest Diet on the Planet
  may contain some salt, sugar, and/or spice.

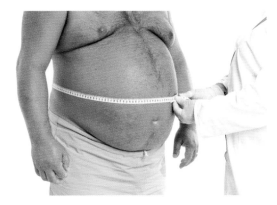

Obesity

Plus complications: hypertension, diabetes, heart disease, cancer, etc.

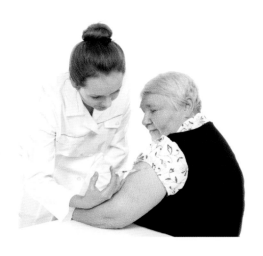

Diabetes

Type 1 and type 2 plus complications: eye damage, kidney failure, gangrene, etc.

"Food Poisoning" Causes

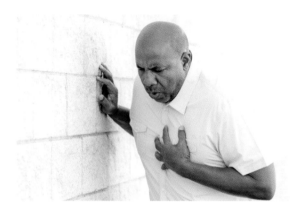

Heart Disease

Heart attacks, strokes, impotence, etc.

"Food Poisoning" Causes

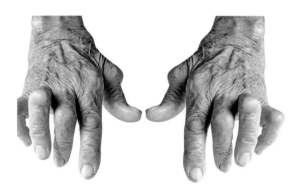

Arthritis

Rheumatoid, psoriatic, lupus, etc.

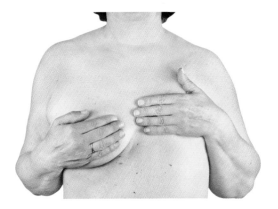

Cancer

Colon, breast, prostate, uterus, etc.

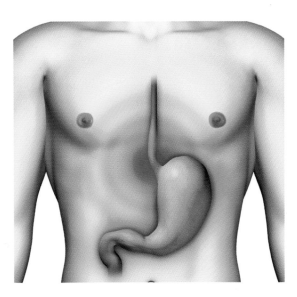

GERD

Indigestion, esophagitis, ulcers, gallbladder disease, etc.

Constipation

Diverticular disease, hemorrhoids, fissures, hiatal hernias, varicose veins, etc.

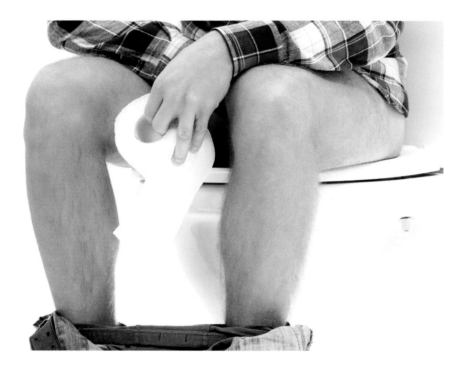

People Are Sick from Eating like Kings and Queens

Historical writings and pictures tell how wealthy people who ate meat, poultry, fish, cheese, eggs, and milk became fat and sick.

The difference is that now billions of people, because of "progress" (the Industrial Revolution and the harnessing of fossil fuels), eat like the aristocrats of the past.

What else would you expect from eating all the rich foods served at Burger King, Dairy Queen, McDonald's, Taco Bell, and KFC, as well as all other restaurants and grocery stores?

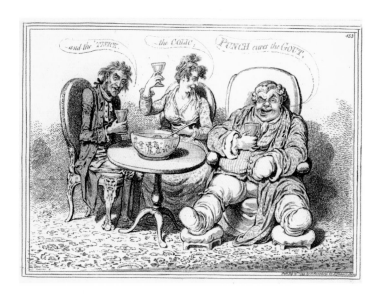

"Food Poisoning"

In order to make this simple, there are two categories of food poisons: animal foods and vegetable oils. After reading this, many people think there is nothing left to eat!

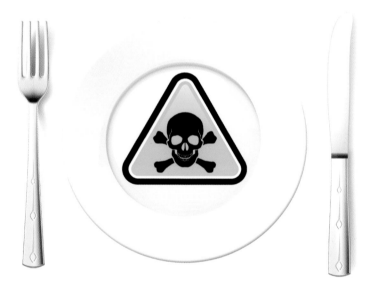

Read on. You will love the foods that make up the Healthiest Diet on the Planet.

Not Food!

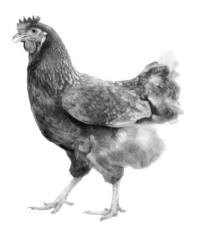

All animal products are full of cholesterol, animal protein, and fat, with no starch, dietary fiber, or other essential sugars for health. They are laced with big doses of people-poisoning environmental chemicals and loads of infection-causing bacteria, parasites, and viruses.

This Is Cat Food!

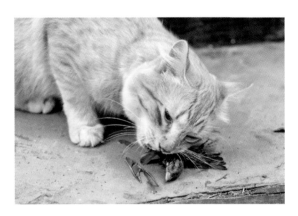

Birds, small mammals, fish, and reptiles are the foods for my cat Einstein, a carnivore. Feeding him baked potatoes instead will result in failure to thrive, followed by death from malnutrition. We are "starchivores" (our diet is, by design, beans, corn, potatoes, and/or rice). Foods ideal for carnivores (meat) or calves (cow's milk) will result in poor health and premature death when consumed by people.

Not Food!

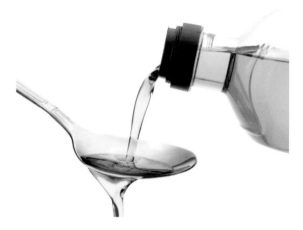

Vegetable oil is an isolated ingredient processed from plants (corn, olives, flaxseeds, etc.). It is calorie dense: 9 calories/gram (compared to sugar at 4 calories/gram, meat and cheese at 4 calories/gram, and starch at 1 calorie/gram). Oil is "empty calories." Bleeding, suppression of the immune system, cancer, and infection are side effects.

A Surefire Cure

Your body is always trying to heal itself.

Simply stop the "food poisoning," and the diseases quickly improve or go away.

"Food poisoning" is primarily caused by eating animal foods and vegetable oils.

One of the Earliest Controlled "Scientific" Trials of the Healthiest Diet on the Planet

A Bible story from 2,600 years ago

Daniel and his men, who ate vegetables, were compared to men who ate animal foods (like most Americans do now). At the end of ten days, the vegetarians looked healthier and better nourished than any of the young men who ate the royal food.

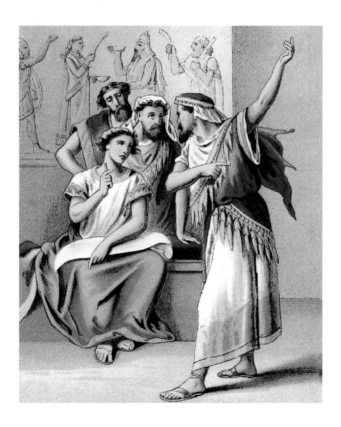

Baha'i faith, nineteenth century

"The food of the future will be fruit and grains. The time will come when meat will no longer be eaten. Medical science is only in its infancy, yet it has shown that our natural food is that which grows out of the ground." Most religions teach the value of grains and other vegetables, and warn about eating meats.

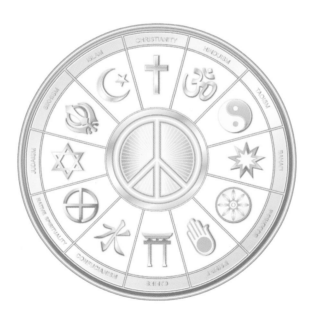

Gladiators Were the "Barley Men"

Strength and endurance come from eating starches.

Think about the warriors of the past and the long-distance runners of today: they are powered by starches. Winners never eat much meat, poultry, dairy, eggs, or oily foods.

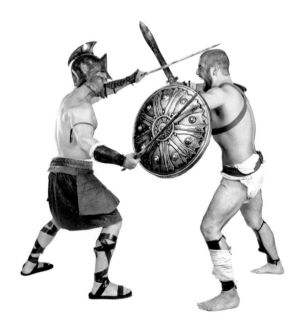

Main Food = Starches

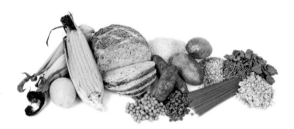

Starches are plant parts that store large amounts of energy for daily activities. They are very low in fat with no cholesterol. They are rich in protein, vitamins, and minerals. Starches are essential for satisfying your appetite, and they make you trim, strong, and healthy.

Eat starch!

Food = Nonstarchy Vegetables

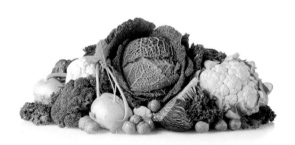

Nonstarchy vegetables provide interest, color, flavor, and some important nutrients (vitamins A and C), but they have insufficient calories to provide for daily energy needs. They should be side dishes only.

You must eat a starch-based diet!

Food = Fruits

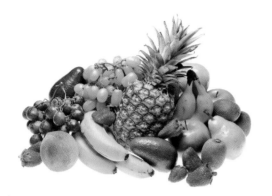

Fruits are mostly simple sugars with some vitamins and minerals. They provide a flavorful (sweet) addition to meals. However, appetite satisfaction is minimal. Generally, one to four fruits daily is a good goal.

You must eat a starch-based diet!

Benefits Happen Quickly

Within twenty-four hours expect relief of constipation, indigestion, GERD, oily skin, and fatigue.

Within four months most chronic problems from "food poisoning" are a matter of history.

This is a cost-free, side-effect-free treatment.

October 14, 2014

McDougall et al. Nutrition Journal 2014, **13**:99
http://www.nutritionj.com/content/13/1/99

NUTRITION
JOURNAL

RESEARCH   **Open Access**

Effects of 7 days on an ad libitum low-fat vegan diet: the McDougall Program cohort

John McDougall[1*], Laurie E Thomas[2], Craig McDougall[3], Gavin Moloney[1], Bradley Saul[4], John S Finnell[5], Kelly Richardson[6] and Katelin Mae Petersen[1]

Abstract

Background: Epidemiologic evidence, reinforced by clinical and laboratory studies, shows that the rich Western diet is the major underlying cause of death and disability (e.g, from cardiovascular disease and type 2 diabetes) in Western industrialized societies. The objective of this study is to document the effects that eating a low-fat (≤10% of calories), high-carbohydrate (~80% of calories), moderate-sodium, purely plant-based diet ad libitum for 7 days can have on the biomarkers of cardiovascular disease and type 2 diabetes.

Methods: Retrospective analysis of measurements of weight, blood pressure, blood sugar, and blood lipids and estimation of cardiovascular disease risk at baseline and day 7 from 1615 participants in a 10-day residential dietary intervention program from 2002 to 2011. Wilcoxon's signed-rank test was used for testing the significance of changes from baseline.

Results: The median (interquartile range, IQR) weight loss was 1.4 (1.8) kg (p < .001). The median (IQR) decrease in total cholesterol was 22 (29) mg/dL (p < .001). Even though most antihypertensive and antihyperglycemic medications were reduced or discontinued at baseline, systolic blood pressure decreased by a median (IQR) of 8 (18) mm Hg (p < .001), diastolic blood pressure by a median (IQR) of 4 (10) mm Hg (p < .001), and blood glucose by a median (IQR) of 3 (11) mg/dL (p < .001). For patients whose risk of a cardiovascular event within 10 years was >7.5% at baseline, the risk dropped to 5.5% (>27%) at day 7 (p < .001).

Conclusions: A low-fat, starch-based, vegan diet eaten ad libitum for 7 days results in significant favorable changes in commonly tested biomarkers that are used to predict future risks for cardiovascular disease and metabolic diseases.

Keywords: Low-fat diet, Vegan diet, Vegetarian diet, Hypertension, Cholesterol, Hyperlipidemia, Type 2 diabetes, Weight loss, Heart disease

Introduction

The primary goal of health care should be to decrease all-cause morbidity and mortality. In industrialized societies including those in the United States and Europe, the chief causes of death and disability are noninfectious chronic diseases: atherosclerotic vascular disease, epithelial cell cancers, type 2 diabetes, and autoimmune disorders [1]. The leading underlying cause of these diseases is the rich Western diet, with its emphasis on animal-source foods (i.e., meat, fish, eggs, and dairy foods) and fat-laden and sugary processed foods [2,3]. These diseases are becoming increasingly prevalent in newly industrialized countries in Central America, South America, and Asia as they, too, adopt Western eating styles [4].

The burden of Western disease can be dramatically reduced by eliminating animal-source foods and vegetable fats from the diet and replacing those foods with low-fat, plant-based foods. When a food rationing system during World War I severely restricted the Danish population's intake of meats, dairy products, fats, and alcohol but placed no restrictions on such foods as barley, bread, potatoes, and vegetables, Denmark achieved the lowest mortality rate in its history [5]. Similarly, the mortality due to diabetes in England and Wales decreased sharply while wartime food rationing in both World War I and World War II limited access to animal-source foods and

* Correspondence: drmcdougall@drmcdougall.com
[1]Dr. McDougall's Health and Medical Center, PO Box 14039, Santa Rosa, CA 95402, USA
Full list of author information is available at the end of the article

Important Medical Findings from Seven Days of Enjoying the Healthiest Diet on the Planet

- The average weight loss was 3.1 pounds while eating unrestricted amounts of food.

- The average cholesterol reduction was 22 mg/dL.

- The average decrease in blood pressure in patients with hypertension (140/90 or greater) was 18/11 mmHg.

- Nearly 90 percent of patients were able to get off blood-pressure and diabetic medications.

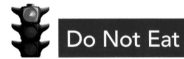

Do Not Eat

Meat

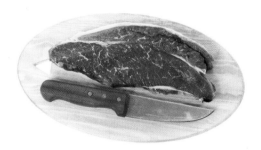

Beef, pork, lamb, deer, buffalo, whale, etc.

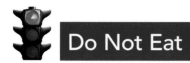

Do Not Eat

Poultry

Chicken, turkey, duck, etc.

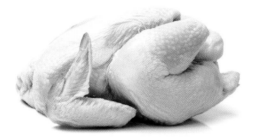

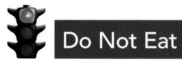

Do Not Eat

Fish

Salmon, tuna, trout, perch, etc.

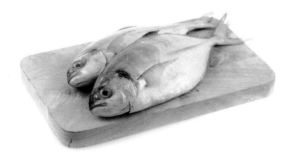

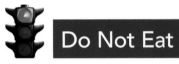

Do Not Eat

Shellfish

Lobster, shrimp, crab, etc.

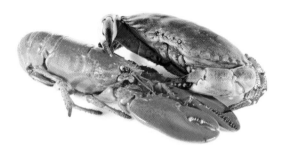

Do Not Eat

Eggs

Chicken, goose, duck, ostrich, etc.

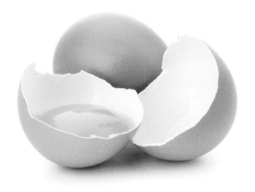

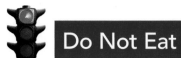

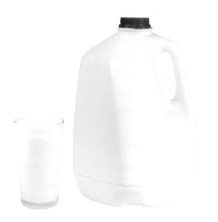

Milk

Cow, goat, sheep, camel, etc.

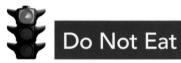 **Do Not Eat**

Cheese

Cow, goat, sheep, camel, etc.

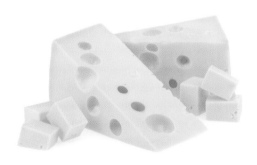

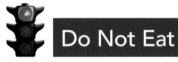

Butter or Margarine

Even all-natural vegan spreads.

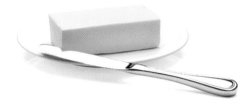

Fake Meats and Cheeses

Hot dogs, sausages, burgers, lunch meats, and nondairy cheeses.

Most are made from isolated proteins from soybeans combined with other chemicals. Also avoid those made from isolated proteins from wheat, peas, fungi, etc.

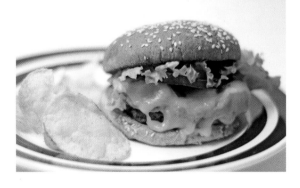

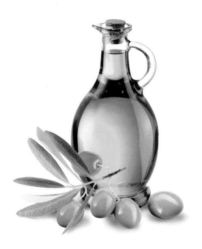

Vegetable Oils

Corn, flaxseed, olive, safflower, etc.

Remember: "The fat (oil) you eat is the fat you wear."

False Advertising in Order to Sell Dangerous Foods

- The meat industries say you must eat their products for protein.

- The dairy industries say their products are necessary for calcium.

- Mention "omega-3 fats" and fish comes to mind immediately.

- The truth is that protein and calcium deficiencies have never been reported on any natural diet sufficient in calories. And only plants can make omega-3 fats; no fish or other animal can make them.

Eat Starches

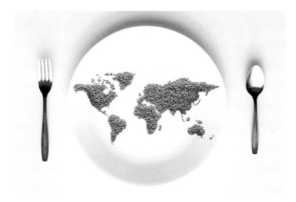

All large populations throughout history ate primarily starch: corn, rice, potatoes, wheat, etc.

Eat Lots Of

Cold Cereal

Wheat, rice, corn, millet, etc.

Use fruit juice or a little rice or soy milk to moisten.

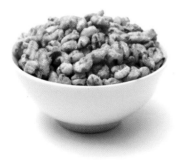

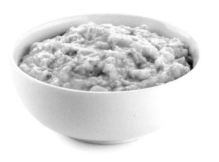

Oatmeal

Millet, kamut, cracked wheat, etc.

You can eat this meal for breakfast, lunch, and/or dinner.

Eat Lots Of

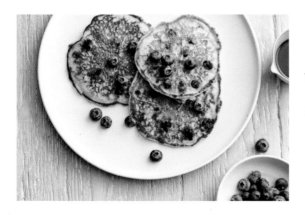

Pancakes

Whole wheat, buckwheat, potato, etc.

No oil, dairy, or eggs.

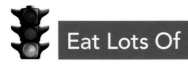

Eat Lots Of

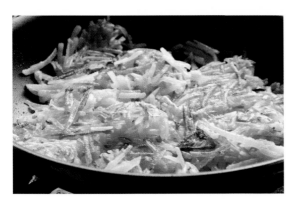

Hash Brown Potatoes

Oil-free. "Fry" in a nonstick pan or on an electric griddle.

Top with salsa, ketchup, or other sauces.

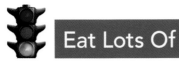

Eat Lots Of

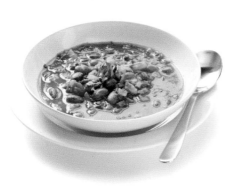

Bean Soups

Minestrone, white bean, pea, lentil, etc.

Cook in slow cooker or pot. Buy already prepared in boxes and cans.

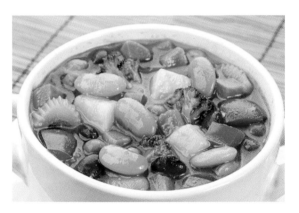

Potato and Carrot Soups

Use your favorite legumes, grains, and vegetables in them.

No animal products or added vegetable oils.

Eat Lots Of

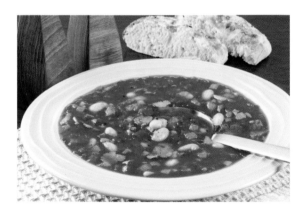

Vegetable Soups

Tomato, onion, corn, celery, broccoli, etc.

Make a big pot and eat all week long with breads, baked potatoes, and other convenient starches.

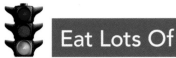

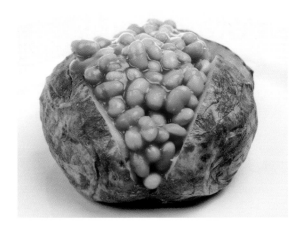

Potatoes

Boiled, baked, or steamed.

Never fried with oil or fat!

Mashed Potatoes

Idaho, Russet, Yukon Gold, etc.

Eat them for breakfast, lunch, and/or dinner.

Potatoes provide complete nutrition, including protein, amino acids, calcium, iron, fiber, and vitamin C.

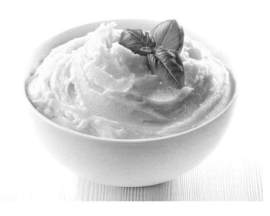

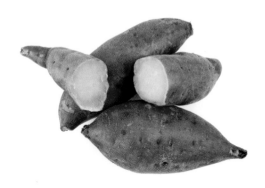

Sweet Potatoes

Baked, mashed, boiled, or steamed.

You can successfully live on a diet of sweet potatoes alone until you find other meals to eat.

Eat Lots Of

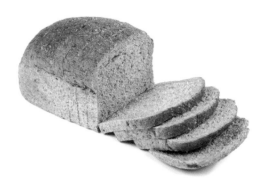

Breads

Whole grain, wheat, rye, etc.

Bread is known as "the staff of life" for good reason.

Do not use butter.

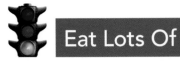

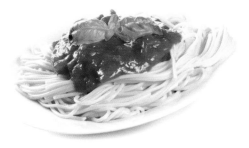

Pastas

Wheat, buckwheat, brown rice, etc.

Think of this as "comfort food."

No olive oil or meat added.

Eat Lots Of

Pizza

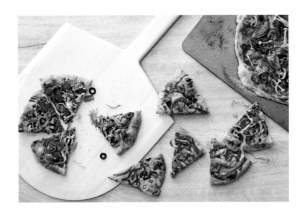

Whole-wheat crust, vegetables, tomato sauce.

Make with your favorite "no oil" sauces and spices.

No cheese or meat.

Brown Rice

And all other whole grains.

Even white rice is better for you than animal foods and vegetable oils.

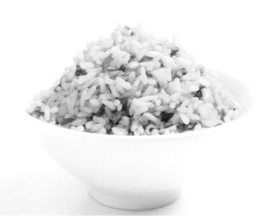

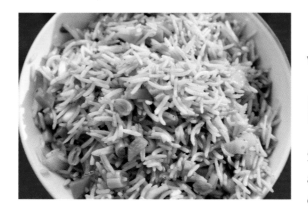

Rice and Vegetable Dishes

Sometimes all you can find is white rice and other refined grain products. Of course, whole-grain is better.

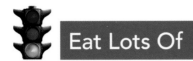

Eat Lots Of

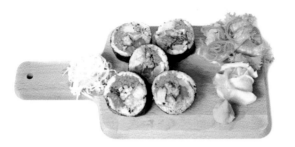

Vegetable Sushi

White rice and white noodles are far better for you than animal foods and vegetable oils.

Look at billions of trim, fit Asians.

Eat Lots Of

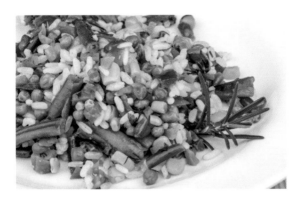

Beans, Rice, and Corn

Eat simple meals of starches, and then add some green vegetables and fruits for vitamins A and C.

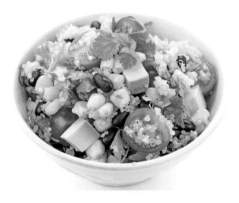

Grain-Based Salads

Bulgur, barley, millet, couscous, quinoa, farro, wheat, rice, etc.

These are traditional Middle Eastern foods.

No vegetable oils, of course.

Eat Lots Of

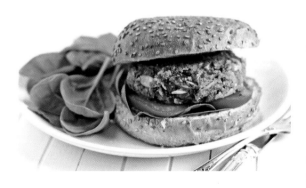

Whole-Grain and Bean-Patty Burgers

No soy burgers.

Garnish with lettuce, tomato, mustard, ketchup, pickle relish, etc.

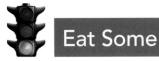
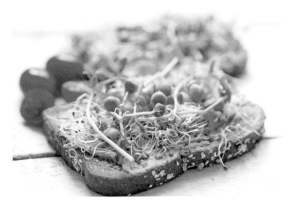

Whole-Grain Bread and Vegetable/Bean-Spread Sandwiches

No fake soy-based meats or cheeses.

Eat Some

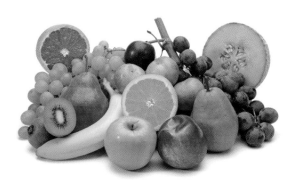

Fruits

Eat one to four a day. Fruits are mostly simple sugars, which offer only a short period of appetite satisfaction—you will be left hungry. These add interest to a starch-based meal plan, but will not sustain you. Starch will satisfy you for a long while!

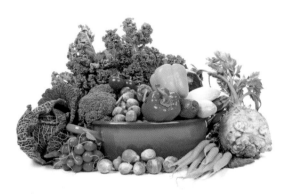

Nonstarchy Vegetables

Eat a few daily. If you eat a diet solely of green, yellow, red, and orange nonstarchy vegetables, you will be hungry all the time.

These foods do add interest and some concentrated nutrients to a starch-based meal plan, but they will not sustain you.

Be Careful

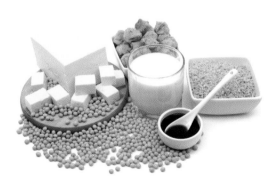

Tofu and Other Natural Soy Products

These are filled with fat. Tofu, miso, soy milk, and other soy products are fine as condiments, but not as the main course.

Remember—no fake meats and cheeses.

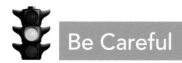

Nuts and Seeds

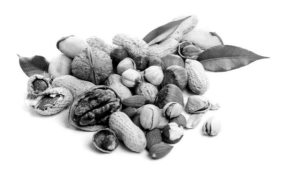

These are filled with fat. They will keep you overweight and obese. You may become a "fat vegan."

Helpful for those in need of gaining weight.

Be Careful

Avocados

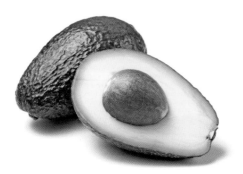

These are filled with fat. Most of the calories (90 percent) are from "good" but fattening fat.

Helpful for those in need of gaining weight.

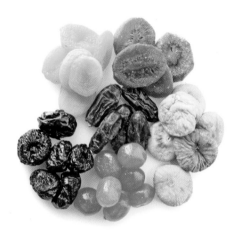

Dried Fruits

Dried fruits are high in simple-sugar calories and provide minimal appetite satisfaction. These "calorie bombs" will slow weight loss.

Helpful for those in need of gaining weight and endurance athletes.

Be Careful

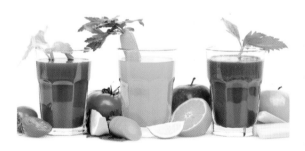

Juices

These are high in simple-sugar calories.

The quality of a food is not improved by beating it a thousand times with a steel blade. This is also true of blending vegetables into juices.

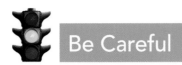

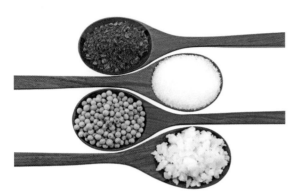

Salt, Sugar, and Spice

Most people can use these for flavor. If in doubt, check with your professional health-care provider.

Do Not Take

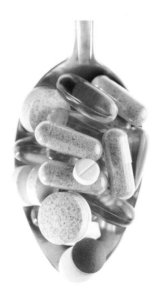

Supplements

Vitamins, minerals, and other plant nutrients are essential for health, but you must get them in their natural packages. Isolated concentrated nutrients found in pills increase your risk of death, heart disease, and cancer.

The only exception is vitamin B12.

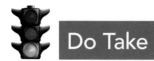

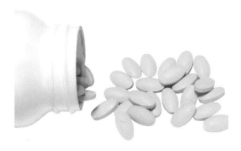

Vitamin B12

The risk of a B12 deficiency disease is extremely small (one in a million) and takes more than three years to develop.

To avoid even a small risk, take this supplement. The need is fewer than 5 micrograms (mcg) daily.

However, the smallest doses sold in stores are 500 mcg. Likely, no side effects occur from the excess. Once a week is adequate.

Sunshine and Exercise

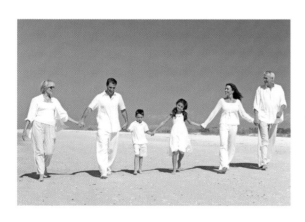

Some Light Exercise

Walking, swimming, bicycling, etc.

Don't hurt yourself with strenuous activities.

Some sunshine is essential (vitamin D and other benefits). *But not too much.*

One Last Thought

If not to save yourself and your family, how about saving Planet Earth?

The livestock industries are producing over half of the global-warming gases, destroying ecosystems, and causing extinction of species. Meat, poultry, egg, dairy, and fish industries are major environmental polluters. Fortunately, we can stop this damage overnight.

Say NO to "food poisoning"!

Instead, eat beans, bread, corn, pasta, potatoes, sweet potatoes, rice, etc.

Please Share This with Others

—John and Mary McDougall
www.drmcdougall.com

5

Recipes for the Healthiest Diet on the Planet

My wife, Mary McDougall, started the low-fat vegan revolution in 1983 with the publication of our first national best-selling book, *The McDougall Plan*. Prior to that the cookbooks on the market were either low-fat *or* vegetarian. The low-fat recipes were focused on lean cuts of beef, skinned chicken, white-meat turkey, egg whites (no yolks), and skim milk–based dairy foods. These foods are unacceptable for the Healthiest Diet on the Planet, because they are very high in animal protein (removing the fat increases the percent of animal protein), causing bone loss and resulting in osteoporosis and kidney stones. Animal foods (even most low-fat versions) are high in cholesterol and have no carbohydrate, dietary fiber, or vitamin C. They are also filthy with environmental contaminants and microbes (bacteria, viruses, and parasites). Following these recipes, artery disease progresses, weight loss is minimal and transient, and constipation and even worse indigestion remain. Environmental damage and animal cruelty continue at the same pace with the "low-fat diet" as with the traditional standard American diet.

Vegetarian cookbooks relied on the heavy use of eggs, dairy products, and vegetable oils back in the 1970s. On our cookbook shelf

Comparison of Macronutrients in Various High- and Low-Fat Foods

(**Note:** percent of calories from protein increases as fat is reduced.)

FOOD	% PROTEIN	% FAT
Egg, whole	35	65
Egg, white	85	15
Milk, whole (3.5%)	21	49
Milk, low-fat (2%)	28	31
Milk, skim	41	2
Turkey, dark	61	39
Turkey, white	80	20

The remainder of the calories from milk are from carbohydrate (lactose); otherwise, animal foods have essentially no carbohydrate.

were *Laurel's Kitchen, Moosewood Cookbook, Diet for a Small Planet,* and *The Vegetarian Epicure.* Even though they avoided eating the living animal, the ingredients contained animal fats and proteins and/ or vegetable fats and were often loaded with cholesterol and contaminants, which would not make them acceptable for the Healthiest Diet on the Planet recipes.

Now it is easy to find vegan recipes, meaning they contain no animal products, but they are heavily laden with vegetable oils, nuts, and seeds, often resulting in meals with more than half of their calories from fat. Sometimes "fake foods," made from isolated soy or wheat proteins, such as soy burgers and faux turkey, are the mainstay of many of the recipes. These chemical concoctions are mixtures of vegetable proteins, vegetable oils, salt, sugars, flavorings, and additives. They are unhealthy. Following these kinds of vegan recipes, people often become "fat vegans" and increase their risk of cancer, type 2 diabetes, gallbladder disease, oily skin, and acne. Fortunately, this vegan approach does positively affect the environment and the horrors of factory farming. However, fat vegans have a difficult time converting others to their important causes (saving the planet and stopping animal cruelty), because their personal appearance is a barrier to communication about the benefits of consuming no animal products.

The transition in diet for us personally came over a period of two years during my internal medicine residency program in Honolulu, Hawaii (1976 to 1978). I would visit the Hawaii State Medical Library and find articles about diet and disease. Quickly I concluded that chicken and fish muscles were the same as the muscles from cows and pigs. Some moved limbs; others flapped wings or swished tails. Initially we decided, "We have to stop all kinds of meat."

"No problem," Mary thought, and she brought out her vegetarian cookbooks and started making recipes centered on milk, cheese, eggs, and vegetable oils.

Further study at the library made me understand that whole dairy and egg products were loaded with saturated fat and cholesterol and had all the same problems as meat. I began referring to cheese as "liquid meat." (The low-fat versions of dairy and eggs have the nutritional problems described above.) Mary's kitchen then became free of animal products.

The next proclamation almost lost me my happy home. I explained, "Vegetable oils are the strongest promoters of cancer of all commonly consumed foods; they make people fat and cause greasy hair and skin. Oils cause bleeding and suppression of the immune system (omega-3), and severe damage to the arteries (omega-6)."

Mary thought, "There is nothing left to cook."

I was busy telling patients the good news about diet; however, they had nothing to eat.

Fortunately, Mary has always been a genius in the kitchen and very dedicated to good health for her family and our patients. Thus the low-fat vegan diet was born. We self-published a ringed notebook/cookbook titled "Making the Change" for our patients, adding more recipes to the binder as Mary and friends invented them.

Mary started an important revolution that has made regaining lost health and personal appearance within reach for everyone. It is

The Macronutrients in Dairy Make It Comparable to Meat				
	GROUND CHUCK	**CHEDDAR CHEESE**	**YOGURT**	**WHOLE MILK**
Percent of calories from fat	68	73	49	50
Percent of calories from protein	32	25	22	21
Percent of calories from carbohydrates	0	2	29	29
Fiber (g)	0	0	0	0
Cholesterol	22	27	21	22
Vitamin C (mg/100 cal)	0	0	0	0

cost-free and side effect–free. On average a family's food expenses are decreased by 60 percent; more, if they had been eating many of their meals out. Medical expenses, including medications, vitamin supplements, doctors' visits, and hospitalizations are eliminated for most.

Currently you can find many vegan recipes with no added vegetable oil and limited use of high-fat nuts, seeds, and avocados by searching the Internet (search for "low-fat vegan" or "fat-free vegan" recipes), and browse your local bookstore or library with the same titles in mind.

Worthwhile Websites

Dr. McDougall's Health & Medical Center, www.drmcdougall.com

Straight Up Food, www.straightupfood.com

Fat-Free Vegan, http://fatfreevegan.com

Happy Herbivore, https://happyherbivore.com

Vegan Coach, www.vegancoach.com

Healthy Girls' Kitchen, www.healthygirlskitchen.com

Engine 2 Diet, http://engine2diet.com

Plant-Powered Kitchen, http://plantpoweredkitchen.com

Low-Fat Vegan Chef, http://lowfatveganchef.com

Cooking with Plants, https://cookingwithplants.com

Plant Based, http://plantbased.org

Vegan Food, http://vegan.food.com

Whole Food Plant Based, www.wholefoodplantbasedrd.com

The Nutrition Professor, http://thenutritionprofessor.com

Plantz Street, https://plantzst.com

Forks Over Knives, www.forksoverknives.com

The main dishes and soups provided in the recipes that follow are based on starches, such as beans, corn, potatoes, rice, and wheat. For the excellent health and personal appearance you desire, the Healthiest Diet on the Planet suggests you consume 70 to 90 percent of your calories from starch. Just "eyeball" your plate, and most of the food should be starch. You should also have some additional nonstarchy green, orange, red, and yellow vegetables (mostly cooked, but some raw foods, such as carrots, celery, kale, lettuce, onions, and peppers make tasty additions).

Mary also provides some delicious desserts that contain some simple sugar. This is not a mistake. Most people can enjoy excellent health even with these occasional special treats (desserts are not the main course). The food is delicious. Add your favorite spices to recipes, and delete any you don't enjoy. When "more taste" is desired, we encourage the addition of small amounts of salt to the surface of the food, where it will be exposed to the salt-sensitive taste buds on the tip of the tongue. Sweet-sensitive flavor buds are also abundant on the tip of the tongue; therefore, a little sugar on your oatmeal and syrup on your pancakes can make all the difference in the enjoyment of your meals. The Healthiest Diet on the Planet is also the Tastiest Diet on the Planet. Mary presents her recipes in the next section. Enjoy!

*Recipes for which there are color photos in the insert are marked with an asterisk (*).

When following a vegan diet (like the Healthiest Diet on the Planet), especially when pregnant or nursing a baby, you should supplement your diet with a minimum of 5 micrograms of vitamin B12 daily.

BREAKFAST

Almond French Toast*

This is a modified version of the French toast that I have been making for many years. This one is even easier, because you don't have to make the almond milk first; you can buy almond milk in aseptic packages in most supermarkets and natural-food stores.

Preparation Time: 5 minutes
Cooking Time: 15 minutes
Servings: 12

---

2 cups almond milk
1 tablespoon brown sugar
⅛ teaspoon cinnamon
Dash turmeric
12 slices whole wheat bread

Combine the almond milk with the brown sugar, cinnamon, and turmeric. (Place in a blender jar and process briefly, use an immersion blender in a deep bowl, or place in a covered jar and shake well.) Dip slices of the bread into this mixture and brown on a medium-hot nonstick griddle. Serve with warmed maple syrup.

Banana Pancakes*

These are a new favorite breakfast in our home. They are easy to make, and everyone loves them! These are wonderful served with a little maple syrup or applesauce. You can make the batter the night before and refrigerate it; just add a bit more liquid to the batter in the morning to thin it.

Preparation Time: 10 minutes
Cooking Time: 10 minutes
Yield: 10 to 12 pancakes

1½ cups unbleached white flour
2 teaspoons baking powder
½ teaspoon salt
1 tablespoon dry egg replacer
1 cup mashed ripe banana (about 2 bananas)
1 cup nondairy milk
1 cup sparkling water
1 cup fresh or frozen blueberries (optional)

Mix the flour, baking powder, salt, and egg replacer in a bowl. Place the mashed banana in another bowl. Stir the nondairy milk and water into the banana and mix well. Pour the banana mixture into the dry ingredients and stir until moistened. Do not overmix! Add the blueberries, if using.

Heat a nonstick griddle over medium heat. Pour about ¼ cup of the batter onto the dry heated griddle and spread slightly with the bottom of your measuring cup. Flip over when the first bubbles start to appear. Cook until brown on both sides. Repeat until all the batter has been used.

Hints: This makes delicious light pancakes that rise as they cook. For a slightly thinner pancake, thin the batter with a little more nondairy milk, stirring it into the mixture well before ladling the batter onto the griddle (the batter thickens if left standing too long before cooking). These may also be made with whole wheat pastry flour, which will result in slightly heavier pancakes.

Breakfast Burritos*

Preparation Time: 10 minutes
Cooking Time: 10 minutes
Servings: 4

1 pound firm water-packed tofu
¼ cup water
¼ cup chopped green onions
¼ cup chopped red bell pepper
1 tablespoon diced canned green chilies
2 teaspoons low-sodium soy sauce
¼ teaspoon turmeric
Pinch crushed red pepper flakes
2 tablespoons chopped fresh cilantro
Mild salsa (optional)
Corn or whole wheat tortillas

Drain the tofu well, mash with a fork, and set aside. Place the water in a nonstick frying pan and add the green onions and red bell pepper. Cook stirring frequently for 3 minutes. Add the mashed tofu, green chilies, soy sauce, turmeric, and red pepper flakes. Continue to cook and stir for another 5 minutes. Stir in the cilantro. Spoon some of this mixture down the center of a warmed tortilla, add salsa, if desired, roll up, and eat.

Hints: This may also be made with firm silken tofu, but the consistency will be much softer. A handful of baby spinach leaves can be added just before the end of the cooking time as a delicious variation. I also like to add some cooked chopped potatoes whenever there are some extras in the refrigerator, adding these at the same time I add the tofu.

Baked French Toast

This is a breakfast that you prepare the evening before, refrigerate overnight, and then just pop into the oven in the morning. After cooking, the French toast is moist on the inside with a slightly crispy top. Serve with warmed maple syrup or a fruit topping (see hints below).

Preparation Time: 5 minutes
Resting Time: Overnight
Cooking Time: 40 minutes
Servings: 6 to 8

9 to 10 slices French or sourdough bread (preferably whole wheat)
4 cups almond milk
3 tablespoons brown sugar
1 teaspoon vanilla
⅛ teaspoon cinnamon
⅛ teaspoon turmeric
⅛ teaspoon salt

Arrange the bread slices in the bottom of two 9 × 13-inch baking dishes. Do not overlap the slices. Place the remaining ingredients in a blender jar and process briefly. Pour over the bread slices in both dishes. Cover and refrigerate overnight.

In the morning, preheat the oven to 350°F.

Remove the covers and bake for about 40 minutes until slightly crisp on the top.

Hints: This is an easy way to make French toast for a crowd without standing over the griddle in the morning. To make a simple fruit sauce, thaw a frozen package of raspberries (or other favorite fruit) overnight in the refrigerator. In the morning, place the thawed fruit in a blender jar, add 1 to 2 tablespoons of agave nectar, and process until smooth.

Sweet Yammy Beginnings

Preparation Time: 5 minutes
Servings: 2

2 *baked* yams or sweet potatoes
2 bananas, peeled and sliced
1 apple, cored and chopped
½ teaspoon cinnamon

Peel and chop the baked yams or sweet potatoes. Combine them with the bananas and apples. Mix in the cinnamon. Heat briefly in a microwave. Serve warm.

Hints: Yams and sweet potatoes may be used interchangeably in this (and most other) recipes. These root vegetables are sold year-round in markets. Sweet potatoes usually are less moist and have pale orange skin and flesh, and the root vegetables usually sold as yams have a reddish skin and deep orange flesh and are usually very moist. This dish may also be served cold or at room temperature.

Gratitude Bowl*

A bowl can be a quick meal if you have some favorite sauces in your refrigerator (see the Sauces section). Simply cook some quinoa or rice, steam a few veggies (frozen are okay also), add some beans or tofu, and top with your favorite sauce. Your choice of ingredients will make this dish different each time you prepare it. Here is my version of a grain and vegetable bowl topped with a simple Tahini Lemon Sauce.

Preparation Time: 15 to 30 minutes
Cooking Time: 15 minutes
Servings: 4

2 tablespoons vegetable broth
1 onion, diced
1 carrot, sliced
¼ pound fresh shiitake mushrooms, stems discarded and caps
    thinly sliced
2 cups broccoli florets
2 cups coarsely chopped kale
1 zucchini, halved lengthwise and sliced
4 to 6 cups *cooked* brown rice or quinoa
1 cup mung bean sprouts
1 avocado, peeled and chopped (optional)

Place the vegetable broth in a large nonstick skillet with the onion and carrots. Cook, stirring occasionally, until the carrot softens slightly, about 5 minutes. Add the mushrooms, cover, and cook until tender, about 4 minutes. Add the broccoli and kale and cook, stirring occasionally, until tender, about 5 more minutes. Add the zucchini and continue to cook until all vegetables are tender, 3 to 5 minutes longer.

Meanwhile, warm the brown rice or quinoa. To serve, place some brown rice, quinoa, or a combination of both, in four large bowls. Top each bowl with some of the cooked vegetable mixture and a few of the mung bean sprouts and avocado chunks. Drizzle a bit of Tahini Lemon Sauce (see the Sauces section) over the top and serve.

Hints: For variation, instead of shiitake, use oyster, cremini, or another of your favorite mushrooms. Instead of the mung bean sprouts, use sunflower sprouts, if you can find them at your local market. Add other vegetables that are in season according to their cooking times.

Incan Bowl

Preparation Time: 15 to 30 minutes
Cooking Time: 15 minutes
Servings: 4

1½ cups uncooked quinoa
3 cups water
6 to 8 cups assorted chopped vegetables (see hints below)
1 to 2 cups sautéed or baked tofu cubes (see hints below)
1½ cups cooked beans of your choice (optional)
Sauce of your choice (see hints below)

Rinse the quinoa well and place it in a pot with the water. Bring to a boil, reduce the heat, cover, and simmer for about 15 minutes, until all the liquid is absorbed.

Steam the vegetables until just tender. Remove them from the heat and place in a bowl.

To serve, place a scoop or two of the quinoa in each of four medium bowls. Layer some of the vegetables over the quinoa, followed by the tofu (and beans, if using). Top it all off with a couple of tablespoons of the sauce of your choice.

Hints: This can be made with any variety of quinoa. Try the red one for a beautiful presentation. Chop the vegetables into similar-sized pieces, so they steam in about the same length of time. Try broccoli, carrots, snow peas, snap peas, broccolini, or asparagus, and don't forget the kale. For tofu cubes, see the recipes in the

Tofu section. Top this with a couple tablespoons of sauce, such as Asian Ginger Sauce, Peanut-Hoisin Sauce, Thai Peanut Sauce, Szechuan Sauce (all in the Sauces section), barbecue sauce, or your favorite oil-free salad dressing. Our favorite variety of this is red quinoa, steamed asparagus, snow peas, lacinato kale, and Asian Marinated Tofu cubes, topped with Peanut-Hoisin Sauce.

Monk Bowl

Preparation Time: 15 to 30 minutes
Cooking Time: 45 minutes
Servings: 4

1½ cups uncooked brown rice
4 cups water
6 to 8 cups assorted chopped vegetables (see hints below)
1 to 2 cups sautéed or baked tofu cubes (see hints below)
1½ cups cooked beans of your choice (optional)
Sauce of your choice (see hints below)

Place the rice and water in a saucepan and bring to a boil. Reduce the heat, cover, and simmer for about 45 minutes until tender.

Steam the vegetables until just tender. Remove from the heat and place in a bowl.

To serve, place a scoop or two of the rice in each of four medium bowls. Layer some of the vegetables over the rice, followed by the tofu (and beans, if using). Top it all off with a couple tablespoons of the sauce of your choice.

Hints: This can be made with any variety of brown rice. Or use instant or frozen brown rice to save time. Chop the vegetables into similar-sized pieces, so they steam in about the same length of time. Try broccoli, carrots, snow peas, snap peas, broccolini, or asparagus, and don't forget the kale. For tofu cubes, see the recipes in the Tofu section. Top this with a couple of tablespoons of sauce, such as an Asian Ginger Sauce, Peanut-Hoisin Sauce, Thai Peanut Sauce, Szechuan Sauce (all in the Sauces section), barbecue sauce, or your favorite oil-free salad dressing. Or turn this into a Korean-style bibimbap by adding some kimchi on top of the vegetables and tofu and mixing some Korean *kochu chang* (or *gochujang*; spicy red pepper paste) into the bowl.

Mayan Bowl

Preparation Time: 15 to 30 minutes

Cooking Time: 15 to 45 minutes

Servings: 4

1½ cups uncooked brown rice or quinoa

4 cups water (3 cups if using quinoa)

2 cups steamed corn

4 cups assorted chopped vegetables

1½ cups cooked beans

Salsa or Enchilada Sauce (see hints below)

Place the rice and water in a saucepan and bring to a boil. Reduce the heat, cover, and simmer for about 45 minutes, until tender. If using quinoa, rinse it well and place it in a pot with the water. Bring to a boil, reduce the heat, cover, and simmer for about 15 minutes, until all the liquid is absorbed.

Steam the vegetables until just tender. Remove from the heat and place in a bowl.

To serve, place a scoop or two of the rice or quinoa in each of four medium bowls. Layer some of the vegetables over the rice or quinoa, followed by the cooked beans of your choice. Top it all off with a couple tablespoons of the sauce of your choice.

Hints: This can be made with any variety of brown rice. Or use instant or frozen brown rice to save some time. Chop the vegetables into similar-sized pieces so they steam in about the same length of time. Try broccoli, carrots, snow peas, snap peas, broccolini, or asparagus, and don't forget the kale. Top this with a couple of tablespoons of sauce, such as fresh salsa or Enchilada Sauce (see the Sauces section).

Ramen Noodle Bowl*

This dish is very easy to put together. Individuals can season their bowl to their liking by adding the amount of hot sauce they prefer.

Preparation Time: 15 minutes
Cooking Time: 10 minutes
Servings: 4

8 cups water
½ cup white miso
⅓ cup Baked Tofu marinade (see hints below)
1 bunch green onions, finely chopped
1 cup sliced mushrooms (see hints below)
1 cup Baked Tofu slices (see hints below)
Ramen noodles (see hints below)
Hot sauce, such as Sriracha (optional)

Place the water in a large pot and bring to a boil. Place the miso in a medium bowl and add 1 to 1½ cups of the boiling water. Whisk until completely smooth. Return to the pan. If you have just made the Baked Tofu recipe, reserve ⅓ cup of the marinade for use in this recipe. Add the reserved marinade to the miso broth. Keep the broth warm, but do not boil.

Meanwhile, prepare the green onions, mushrooms, and tofu and set them aside in separate bowls. Bring another large pot of water to a boil, drop in the ramen noodles, and cook until just tender, 3 to 5 minutes depending on which kind was used (see hints below).

Place an equal amount of noodles in each of four large soup bowls. Ladle the broth over the noodles and top each bowl with equal amounts of green onions, mushrooms, and baked tofu. Serve with Sriracha or other hot sauce on the side for each person to add as desired.

Hints: Use some exotic mushrooms in this recipe if you can find them at your market, such as oyster, chanterelles, or enoki; however, sliced white or cremini are also delicious.

Make the Baked Tofu (see the Tofu section) ahead of time and reserve the rest for snacking or another recipe. Save the extra marinade for use in this recipe.

Ramen noodles are made from wheat flour, water, and salt. Be sure to read the ingredients carefully, as some products do contain eggs. The widest variety of noodles will be found in large Asian markets. Follow the directions for cooking time on the package. Fresh noodles will take less time to cook than dried noodles. Annie Chun's makes fresh packs of organic noodles that are available in many markets. They just need to be dropped into boiling water and are softened and ready to use in recipes in 3 minutes. They come 2 packs to a package, and each pack weighs 6 ounces already cooked. I use 4 packs in the recipe above.

Creamy Corn Soup

This soup is wonderful as a first course, as it may be served warm or at room temperature. It is delicious plain or with a dollop of Tofu Chili Cream (see the Sauces section) for a bit more heat and flavor.

Preparation Time: 10 minutes
Cooking Time: 15 minutes
Servings: 6

4¼ cups vegetable broth, *divided*
1 small mild onion, chopped
2 tablespoons unbleached white flour
1 to 2 tablespoons canned chopped green chilies
4 cups frozen corn kernels, thawed
1 tablespoon chopped fresh cilantro

Place ¼ cup of the broth in a medium saucepan. Add the onions and cook and stir for 2 to 3 minutes. Stir in the flour and mix well. Add the remaining broth, about ¼ cup at a time, stirring well, until the flour is mixed into the broth. Stir in the green chilies and the corn and heat the soup to boiling. Reduce the heat and cook for about 5 minutes. Remove by cupfuls to a blender jar and process briefly until slightly smooth. Return the soup to the pan and heat through. Stir in the cilantro just before serving. Serve warm or at room temperature.

Beans and Greens Soup

This soup is quick to put together with staples from your pantry and refrigerator. It can be easily varied according to what you have on hand. See the hints below for some suggestions. Since we tend to like our food spicy, I usually serve this with hot pepper sauce to shake over the top. And of course slices of hearty bread to dunk in the broth.

Preparation Time: 15 minutes
Cooking Time: 20 minutes
Servings: 6

1 onion, chopped
1 stalk celery, chopped
1 carrot, chopped
5 cups vegetable broth, *divided*
1 teaspoon minced fresh garlic
1 tablespoon low-sodium soy sauce
Dash red pepper flakes
6 cups chopped greens
3 (15-ounce) cans beans, drained and rinsed
1 tablespoon red wine vinegar
Freshly ground black pepper to taste
Hot sauce, such as Sriracha (optional)

Place the onion, celery, and carrot in a large soup pot with ¼ cup of the vegetable broth. Cook, stirring occasionally, for about 5 minutes, until the vegetables soften slightly. Stir in the garlic and soy sauce. Add 4 cups of the vegetable broth, the red pepper flakes, the greens, and 3 cups of the cooked beans. Bring to a boil, reduce the heat, and simmer until the greens are tender, about 10 minutes. Place the remaining beans and broth in a blender jar and process until smooth. Add to the soup pot. Add the vinegar and black pepper to taste. Heat through, and serve with the hot sauce, if desired.

Hints: We like this best with hearty greens, such as kale or Swiss chard. Make this with a variety of beans for a more colorful soup; different beans will give this soup different flavors and textures. Try it with 2 cans of white beans (blend one of them in a blender) and 1 can of red or black beans. Or try this with garbanzo beans. One can of diced tomatoes may also be added to this soup, or try adding 1 to 2 tablespoons tomato paste to the processed bean mixture.

Beany Minestrone Soup*

This soup uses refried beans as a thickener, so the resulting soup is very thick and rich without having to cook all day. Since I almost always have some leftover smashed pinto beans in my refrigerator, I decided to incorporate them into my version of this delicious soup.

Preparation Time: 20 minutes
Cooking Time: 1 hour
Servings: 8

1 onion, chopped
2 teaspoons minced fresh garlic
2 stalks celery, sliced
2 carrots, sliced
6½ cups vegetable broth, *divided*
1 (14.5-ounce) can fire-roasted diced tomatoes
1 (8-ounce) can tomato sauce
6 to 8 fingerling potatoes, sliced
1½ cups fat-free refried beans
1 bay leaf
2 tablespoons parsley flakes
1½ teaspoons dried basil
1½ teaspoons dried oregano
Freshly ground black pepper
1 (15-ounce) can kidney beans, drained and rinsed
¾ cup frozen corn kernels
½ cup uncooked whole wheat pasta elbows
2 cups chopped Swiss chard
1 teaspoon balsamic vinegar

Place the onions, garlic, celery, and carrots in a large pot with ½ cup of the vegetable broth. Cook, stirring frequently, for about 5 minutes, until the onions are softened. Add the remaining broth, tomatoes, tomato sauce, potatoes, refried beans, bay leaf, parsley, basil, oregano, and black pepper. Bring to a boil, reduce the heat, cover, and simmer for 25 minutes, stirring occasionally to smooth out the refried beans. Add the kidney beans, corn, and whole wheat elbows. Continue to cook for 20 minutes. Stir in the chard and balsamic vinegar and cook an additional 10 minutes until the chard is softened. Remove the bay leaf before serving.

Hint: If you do not have leftover beans in your refrigerator, substitute 1 (15-ounce) can of fat-free refried beans.

Fresh Tomato Gazpacho

There are many varieties of gazpacho: white, red, yellow, and green; Spanish, Mexican, Tex-Mex, and Italian; and even fruit-based gazpachos. The word *gazpacho* translates into English as "salad soup," and what better way to describe this refreshing veggie delight? It's generally acknowledged that gazpacho got its start in the Andalusian area of Spain, where the warm Mediterranean summers are balanced by cool food choices. But it was in the Americas that tomatoes were first added to this dish to create the widely popular red gazpacho.

Preparation Time: 35 minutes
Cooking Time: 13 minutes
Chilling Time: 3 hours
Servings: 6 to 8

1 pound mushrooms, cut in half, then sliced
½ cup vegetable broth or water, *divided*
¼ cup low-sodium soy sauce
¾ cup thinly sliced onion wedges, separated
8 tomatoes, chopped (reserve as much juice as you can)
1 tablespoon lime juice
½ cup ketchup
1½ cups hearts of palm, chopped (1 14.5-ounce can, drained)
½ cup chopped fresh cilantro
Freshly ground black pepper
Hot sauce (optional)

Place the mushrooms in a large nonstick frying pan with ¼ cup of the vegetable broth or water and the soy sauce. Cook over medium heat, stirring occasionally, for 5 minutes. Remove the mushrooms from the heat, drain, reserving the liquid, and set aside in a large bowl.

Place the remaining ¼ cup of the vegetable broth or water in the frying pan with the onion. Cook over medium heat, stirring occasionally, for about 3 minutes, until the onions are translucent and most of the liquid has evaporated. Remove from the heat and add to the mushrooms.

Place the tomatoes and their juice in the frying pan with the lime juice and ketchup. Cook over medium heat, stirring occasionally, for 5 minutes. Remove from the heat and add to the mushrooms and onions. Add the hearts of palm and cilantro. Mix well, cover, and refrigerate at least 3 hours to allow the flavors to blend.

Before serving, taste the chilled soup and add several twists of freshly ground black pepper, hot sauce to taste, and 2 to 3 tablespoons of the reserved liquid from cooking the mushrooms.

Hint: This is even better if you can refrigerate it for 24 hours before serving.

Hearty Garbanzo Soup

I tend to focus on soups at the beginning of fall since they are easy to prepare and serve, and are very satisfying to eat. Cleanup is also easy! Whenever I have a large assortment of fresh herbs growing in my garden, I take advantage of them by adding them to this soup.

Preparation Time: 20 minutes
Cooking Time: 60 minutes
Servings: 4 to 6

1 onion, chopped
1 teaspoon minced fresh garlic
4 cups vegetable broth
1 pound mushrooms, sliced
1½ cups shredded green cabbage
1 teaspoon ground cumin
¼ teaspoon ground coriander
1 (15-ounce) can garbanzo beans, undrained
1 (15-ounce) can garbanzo beans, drained and rinsed
2 tablespoons tahini
¾ cup jarred roasted red bell pepper strips
1 to 2 teaspoons chili-garlic sauce
½ cup chopped fresh parsley
¼ cup chopped fresh cilantro
¼ cup chopped fresh dillweed
¼ cup chopped fresh chives
2 tablespoons lemon juice
Dash sea salt

Place the onion and garlic in a large soup pot with about 1 tablespoon of the vegetable broth. Cook, stirring frequently, until the onion softens and turns translucent. Add the remaining vegetable broth and bring to a boil. Add the mushrooms, cabbage, cumin, and coriander. Cover and simmer for about 15 minutes.

Meanwhile, pour the undrained can of garbanzo beans into a blender jar. Add the tahini and process until smooth. Add the processed beans and the can of drained and rinsed beans to the soup pot as well as the roasted red pepper strips and the chili-garlic sauce. Slowly bring to a boil, reduce the heat, cover, and simmer for 45 minutes. Add the fresh herbs and lemon juice and simmer for an additional 15 minutes. Season with a bit of sea salt before serving, if desired.

Moroccan Harira

This delicious soup is made with common brown-green lentils and canned tomatoes, which are readily available. This is a very thick, hearty stew, which is delicious on a cool fall evening with slices of fresh bread.

Preparation Time: 15 minutes
Cooking Time: 1 hour
Servings: 8

1 onion, chopped
2 stalks celery, chopped
2 cloves fresh garlic, crushed
8 cups vegetable broth
1 (14.5-ounce) can diced tomatoes
1 (15-ounce) can garbanzo beans, drained and rinsed
1 cup dried brown-green lentils
1 tablespoon tomato paste
1 tablespoon lemon juice
½ teaspoon cinnamon
½ teaspoon paprika
½ teaspoon ground ginger
½ teaspoon ground coriander
½ teaspoon ground turmeric
¼ teaspoon ground nutmeg
¼ teaspoon freshly ground black pepper
⅛ teaspoon ground cloves
½ cup orzo (rice-shaped pasta)
2 tablespoons chopped fresh cilantro
2 tablespoons chopped fresh flat-leaf parsley

Place the onion, celery, and garlic in a large soup pot with about 2 tablespoons of vegetable broth. Cook, stirring frequently, until the vegetables become slightly softened. Add the remaining vegetable broth, tomatoes, garbanzo beans, lentils, tomato paste, lemon juice, and all of the spices to the pot. Mix well, bring to a boil, reduce the heat, cover, and cook for about 40 minutes, until the lentils are tender. Add the orzo and cook for another 15 minutes. Stir in the fresh cilantro and parsley and serve at once.

Mexican Bean Soup

This is an easy soup that anyone can put together with very little effort for delicious results! The optional chipotle chili powder adds a smoky flavor and a bit more heat to the soup.

Preparation Time: 5 minutes
Cooking Time: 30 minutes
Servings: 6

1 (32-ounce) box vegetable broth
1 onion, chopped
1 teaspoon minced fresh garlic
2 teaspoons ground cumin
1 teaspoon ground oregano
2 cups frozen corn kernels
2 (15-ounce) cans black beans, drained and rinsed
2 (14.5-ounce) cans fire-roasted diced tomatoes with green chilies
⅛ teaspoon chipotle chili powder (optional)

Place ¼ cup of the broth in a large saucepan. Add the onion and garlic and cook for about 4 minutes, stirring frequently. Add the cumin and oregano and stir for another minute. Then add the remaining broth, corn, beans, tomatoes, and chipotle chili powder, if using. Bring to a boil, reduce the heat, cover, and cook over low heat for about 20 minutes.

Soba Miso Soup

This delicious version of miso soup is a bit heartier with the addition of buckwheat soba noodles.

Preparation Time: 10 minutes
Cooking Time: 5 minutes
Resting Time: 5 minutes
Servings: 4

6 cups water
⅓ cup white miso
2 tablespoons soy sauce
1 (12.3-ounce) package firm silken tofu, cubed
12 ounces cooked buckwheat soba noodles (see hints below)
1 cup packed baby spinach
1 bunch green onions, chopped
¼ teaspoon red pepper flakes

Place the water in a large pot and bring to a boil. Remove about ¾ cup of the water and place in a bowl with the miso. Whisk until very smooth. Return the mixture to the pot and add the remaining ingredients. Heat through for 1 to 2 minutes, then turn off the heat, cover, and let rest for about 5 minutes.

Hints: Using cooked buckwheat soba noodles, which are available in some markets, saves a bit of preparation time. If you cannot find precooked soba noodles, use about 4 ounces of dried soba noodles and cook according to package directions before using in this recipe.

Split Pea Soup

This pea soup is a favorite with all of my grandsons. I start it cooking in the morning when I hear they are coming over for the day, and they snack on it all afternoon. It tastes even better the next day and is great over baked potatoes too!

Preparation Time: 15 minutes
Cooking Time: 2 hours
Servings: 8 to 10

2 cups dried green split peas
¼ cup barley
8 cups water
2 bay leaves
1 teaspoon celery seed
1 onion, chopped
2 carrots, chopped
2 potatoes, peeled and cubed
2 celery stalks, chopped
2 tablespoons parsley flakes
1 teaspoon dried basil
Freshly ground black pepper to taste

Place split peas, barley, and water in a large pot. Bring to a boil, reduce heat, and add the bay leaves and celery seed. Cover and cook over low heat for 30 minutes. Add the remaining ingredients and cook for 1 additional hour.

Hints: This freezes and reheats well. To save some potato-peeling and -chopping time, use oil-free cubed hash brown potatoes, about 1 cup.

Marinated Sautéed Tofu

I prefer to marinate and dry-sauté (or dry-fry) my own tofu, because it tastes so much better than the baked tofu that is available in markets. This method results in slightly crispy cubes that can be used in a variety of dishes.

Preparation Time: 5 minutes
Marinating Time: 10 minutes
Cooking Time: 10 minutes
Servings: variable

> 1 (10-ounce) package extra-firm tofu
> 2 tablespoons low-sodium soy sauce
> 1 tablespoon agave nectar
> Dash sesame oil (optional)

Drain the tofu well, cut it into cubes, and place it in a large bowl. Mix the soy sauce, agave nectar, and sesame oil together. Pour this mixture over the tofu cubes and stir well. Let the cubes marinate for about 10 minutes, stirring occasionally to make sure they are well coated. Remove the tofu from the marinade with a slotted spoon and dry-fry it in a nonstick skillet until nicely browned on all sides, turning occasionally with a spatula.

Asian Marinated Tofu

Preparation Time: 5 minutes
Marinating Time: 30 minutes
Cooking Time: 10 minutes
Servings: variable

20 ounces extra-firm tofu
2 tablespoons rice vinegar
2 tablespoons light miso
1 tablespoon low-sodium soy sauce
1 tablespoon tahini
1 tablespoon agave nectar
2 teaspoons mirin

Drain the tofu and cut it into small cubes.

Place the remaining ingredients in a small bowl and whisk until smooth. Pour this over the tofu and toss to coat well. Let the tofu marinate for at least 30 minutes, tossing occasionally to make sure the tofu is well saturated.

Place the tofu cubes along with the marinade in a large nonstick sauté pan. Dry-fry the cubes for about 10 minutes, turning occasionally with a spatula to make sure the cubes are well browned on all sides.

Baked Tofu

Preparation Time: 5 minutes
Marinating Time: 10 minutes
Cooking Time: 25 to 30 minutes
Servings: variable

20 ounces extra-firm tofu
¼ cup low-sodium soy sauce
2 tablespoons rice vinegar
1 teaspoon agave nectar
Dash sesame oil (optional)

Drain the tofu and cut it into ¼-inch slices. Place them in a large flat baking dish. Combine the remaining ingredients and pour over the tofu slices. Allow the tofu to marinate for at least 10 minutes and up to 1 hour. (Or place it in the refrigerator and marinate overnight.)

Preheat the oven to 375°F.

Remove the tofu slices from the marinade and place them on a nonstick baking sheet. Bake for 25 to 30 minutes, turning once halfway through the baking time. They should be brown and crispy on the outside when done. Remove from the oven and cool. Slice into strips or cubes for use in recipes calling for baked tofu.

Hints: This tastes much better (and is less expensive and healthier) than the baked tofu found in packages in many markets and natural-food stores. Other seasonings may be added as desired, such as garlic, ginger, balsamic vinegar, or rosemary, to enhance the flavor of the tofu. It's also delicious just marinated in plain soy sauce. The marinade may be saved for later use in a covered jar in the refrigerator for a couple of weeks. The tofu may also be cubed before baking, resulting in slightly crispier cubes.

Asian Pasta Salad

This salad is a favorite with our grandsons Jaysen and Ben.

Preparation Time: 20 minutes
Cooking Time: 15 minutes
Chilling Time: 2 hours
Servings: 4

½ pound buckwheat soba noodles
½ cup water
4 tablespoons low-sodium soy sauce, *divided*
2 cloves garlic, crushed
1 teaspoon grated fresh ginger
¼ teaspoon red pepper flakes
4 cups broccoli florets
2 carrots, sliced
½ pound mushrooms, sliced
1 bunch green onions, cut into 1-inch pieces
1 tablespoon cornstarch mixed in 2 tablespoons cold water

Prepare the soba noodles according to package directions. Drain. Toss with 2 tablespoons of the soy sauce and set aside.

Meanwhile, place the water, 2 tablespoons of the soy sauce, the garlic, ginger, and red pepper flakes in a wok or large sauté pan. Bring to a boil, add the broccoli and carrots, and cook, stirring frequently, for 5 minutes. Add the mushrooms and green onions and continue to cook, stirring frequently, for about 7 minutes, until the broccoli is tender. Stir in the cornstarch mixture and cook, stirring, until thickened. Pour over the soba noodles and toss to mix well. Refrigerate for at least 2 hours for best flavor. Serve cold.

Barbecued Bean Salad

This delicious salad is easy to prepare and can be served in many different ways. It can be eaten plain as a side dish, as a topping for chilled greens (such as spinach or lettuce), stuffed into pita bread with some fresh chopped greens, or rolled up in a wrap by itself or with barbecued tofu or greens.

Preparation Time: 15 minutes
Chilling Time: 2 hours
Servings: 4 to 6

1 (15-ounce) can black beans, drained and rinsed
1 (15-ounce) can pinto beans, drained and rinsed
1 (15-ounce) can white beans, drained and rinsed
½ cup diced sweet onion
1 stalk celery, diced
1 medium red bell pepper, diced
1 cup frozen corn kernels, thawed
½ cup bottled oil-free barbecue sauce
1 tablespoon red wine vinegar
2 teaspoons Dijon mustard
Dash salt

Place the beans in a large bowl. Add the vegetables and mix well. Add the remaining ingredients and toss again to mix. Refrigerate to blend flavors.

Hints: To use home-cooked beans in this recipe, cook your beans in a pressure cooker or on the stove and use about 1½ cups cooked beans for each can of beans called for. This may also be made with other varieties of beans; choose all one kind or a mixture of different beans. To use fresh corn instead of frozen, cook two ears of corn until tender. Cool. Slice the kernels from the cob and use as directed above.

Border Salad*

Make this salad ahead of time to allow the flavors to become bolder. This is delicious in a bowl as a refreshing summer meal. Or serve this on top of a plate of assorted greens or bowl of cooked grains, rolled up in a tortilla, or as a topping for baked potatoes.

Preparation Time: 20 minutes
Chilling Time: 2 to 4 hours
Servings: 6 to 8

2 (15-ounce) cans kidney beans, drained and rinsed
1 small red onion, chopped
4 stalks celery, chopped
1 green bell pepper, chopped
1 cup baby corns, cut in half
1 cup sliced roasted red bell peppers (see hints below)
1 (14-ounce) can water-packed hearts of palm, drained and sliced
1 (15-ounce) can water-packed artichoke hearts, drained and cut in half
1 medium or large tomato, chopped
1 small jalapeño pepper, seeded and chopped (optional)
¼ cup chopped fresh cilantro
1½ cups fresh salsa (see hints below)

Place all the ingredients except the salsa in a large bowl and mix well. Process the salsa in a blender jar until fairly smooth and pour over the vegetable mixture. Toss to mix. Cover and refrigerate for 2 to 4 hours to allow the flavors to blend.

Hints: You may either buy jarred roasted red bell peppers (just be sure they are not packed in oil) or roast your own. Blending the salsa makes for a smoother Mexican-style dressing for this salad. If you like your dressing a bit chunkier, just add it to the vegetables without blending. The jalapeño does give this salad some heat, so feel free to omit it, if desired. For those of you who don't like cilantro, just leave it out or substitute parsley instead. This salad will keep in the refrigerator for several days.

Crunchy Quinoa Salad*

Feel free to vary the vegetables in this salad according to what you have in your garden or find at the farmers' market.

Preparation Time: 30 minutes
Chilling Time: 1 to 2 hours
Servings: 6

---

1 cup uncooked quinoa
2 cups vegetable broth
3 2-inch strips of lemon zest (see hints below)
1½ cups asparagus, sliced into ½-inch pieces
1 cup snow peas, cut in half
½ cup kohlrabi, peeled and sliced into thin strips
⅓ cup thinly sliced radishes
3 tablespoons lemon juice
2 tablespoons chopped fresh chives
2 tablespoons chopped fresh parsley
1 tablespoon chopped fresh cilantro (optional)
1 teaspoon chopped fresh mint
Freshly ground black pepper
Dash sea salt

Rinse the quinoa well and place it in a pot with the vegetable broth and bring to a boil. Reduce the heat, stir in the pieces of lemon zest, cover, and cook for 15 minutes. Remove from the heat, stir, and remove and discard the pieces of lemon zest. Allow the quinoa to cool slightly.

Meanwhile, put a large pot of water on the stove to boil, drop the asparagus and snow peas into the boiling water, and cook for 2 to 3 minutes, until crisp-tender (do not overcook; the vegetables should still be slightly firm). Remove from the pot with a slotted spoon and drop into a bowl of ice water. Drain.

Combine the cooked quinoa, asparagus, snow peas, kohlrabi, and radishes in a large bowl. Add the remaining ingredients and mix well. Season with freshly ground black pepper and sea salt, if desired. Chill for 1 to 2 hours before serving to allow flavors to mingle.

Hints: Peel the lemon with a vegetable peeler, yielding very thin strips. Use the remaining lemon for the juice in this recipe. Kohlrabi, a relative of cabbage and broccoli, may be unfamiliar to you, but I highly recommend it in this recipe. If you can't find it, use sliced zucchini instead.

Green Goddess Potato Salad

I saw a recipe for a simple green potato salad in a magazine a couple of months ago and the photo was so appealing that I decided to try something similar—without the mayonnaise and sour cream, of course. I made this with only potatoes, but if you like other chopped vegetables (such as celery or onion) in your potato salad, feel free to add them.

Preparation Time: 20 minutes
Cooking Time: 15 minutes
Chilling Time: 2 to 4 hours
Servings: 4 to 8

4 pounds red potatoes

DRESSING

1 (12.3-ounce) package soft silken tofu
¼ cup water
2 tablespoons white wine vinegar
2 tablespoons lime juice
2 tablespoons tahini
2 tablespoons low-sodium soy sauce
½ tablespoon white miso
1 bunch green onions, chopped
1 cup chopped fresh flat-leaf parsley
Freshly ground black pepper

For the dressing, place the tofu and water in a blender jar and process briefly. Add the remaining dressing ingredients and process until very smooth and green. Set aside.

Scrub the potatoes, but do not peel them. Cut them into approximately 1-inch chunks. Place the potatoes in a pot with water to cover. Bring to a boil, reduce the heat, and cook for about 12 minutes, until just tender. Drain. Allow the potatoes to cool for 15 minutes.

Place the cooled potatoes in a large bowl. Add any other chopped vegetables if you wish at this time. Pour 1½ cups of the dressing over the potatoes and mix gently. Cover and refrigerate at least 2 hours before serving.

Hint: Reserve the remaining dressing for use later as a dip for raw veggies or a topping for salad greens.

Israeli Couscous Salad

Israeli couscous can be found in most supermarkets in the ethnic-foods section. It looks like large couscous. If you are unable to find it, another small pasta (like orzo or small shells) may be substituted. Follow directions for cooking time on the individual package.

Preparation Time: 15 minutes
Chilling Time: 60 minutes
Servings: 4

4 cups *cooked* Israeli couscous
1 cup frozen corn kernels, thawed
½ cup chopped green onions
½ cup diced red pepper
½ cup diced yellow pepper
½ cup minced fresh parsley
¼ cup pitted and chopped black olives
¾ cup fat-free dressing (see hints below)
1 teaspoon low-sodium soy sauce
¼ to ½ teaspoon chopped fresh dillweed
Dash Tabasco sauce
Freshly ground black pepper

Place the cooked couscous in a large bowl. Add all the vegetables and mix well. Combine the dressing, soy sauce, dillweed, and Tabasco. Pour this over the salad mixture and toss to mix. Season with pepper to taste. Chill before serving.

Hints: This is delicious with many different kinds of dressing. Try fat-free Italian, honey-mustard, raspberry vinaigrette, sesame, or your favorite dressing. This keeps well in the refrigerator, and it is easy to pack for a lunch on the go. It is one of my favorite salads, and I usually make a double batch.

POTATO, RICE, BEAN, AND PASTA DISHES

Asian Vegetable Noodle Toss*

This is a delicious soba noodle and vegetable toss. The vegetables can easily be varied to suit your taste or the availability of produce. It may be served warm or at room temperature.

Preparation Time: 30 minutes
Cooking Time: 20 minutes
Servings: 3 to 4

---

1 pound asparagus, trimmed and cut into 1-inch pieces
1½ cups trimmed and halved snow peas
1 cup Marinated Sautéed Tofu cubes (see hint below)
9.5 ounces buckwheat soba noodles
1 tablespoon low-sodium soy sauce

ASIAN SAUCE

2 tablespoons low-sodium soy sauce
1 tablespoon mirin
½ tablespoon agave nectar
½ tablespoon rice vinegar
1 clove garlic, crushed
2 teaspoons cornstarch mixed in 1 tablespoon cold water
Dash sesame oil or chili oil (optional)
Pinch crushed red pepper flakes (optional)

Put a large pot of water on to boil. Add the vegetables to the boiling water and cook for about 2 minutes. Remove the vegetables from the water with a strainer and place them in a large bowl. Add the tofu and mix well.

Bring the water back to a boil. Add the soba noodles and cook for 4 to 5 minutes, until tender.

For the Asian Sauce place all the sauce ingredients in a saucepan. Slowly bring to a boil, stirring constantly, until thickened and clear. Remove from the heat and pour over the tofu and vegetables, mixing well.

Remove soba noodles from water and place in a large bowl. Toss with the 1 tablespoon soy sauce to separate the noodles. Pour the vegetable mixture over the noodles and toss well to mix. Serve warm or at room temperature, with Sriracha hot sauce as a condiment, if desired, for more heat.

Hint: For the Marinated Sautéed Tofu cubes, see the Tofu section.

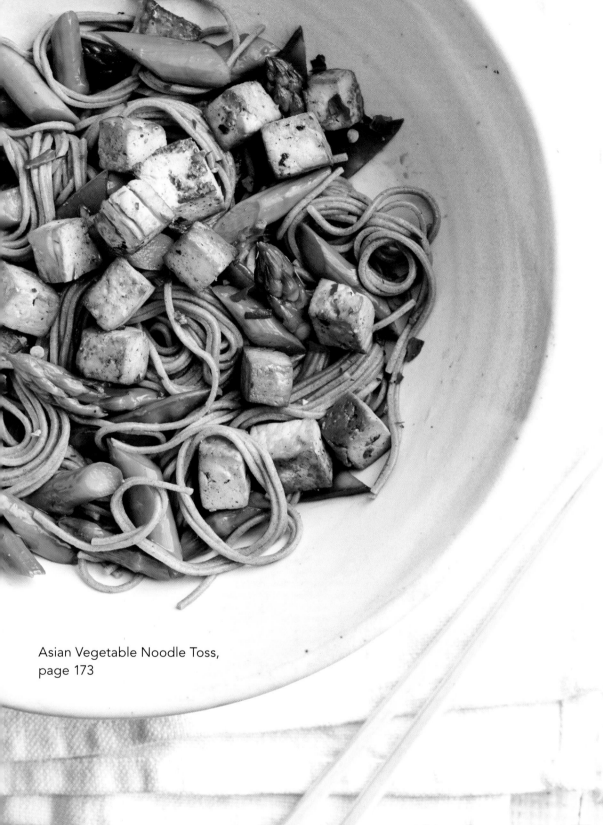

Asian Vegetable Noodle Toss,
page 173

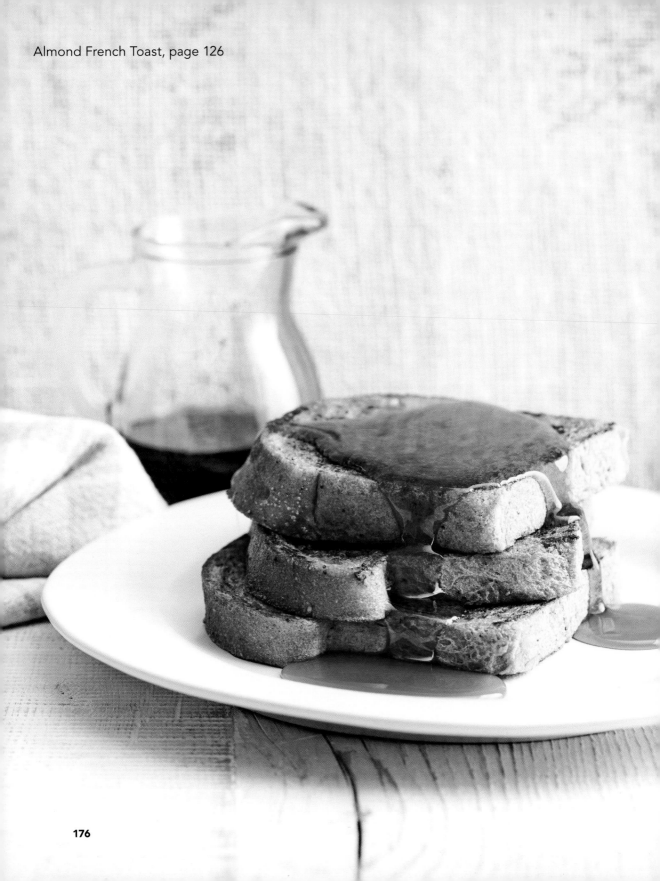

Almond French Toast, page 126

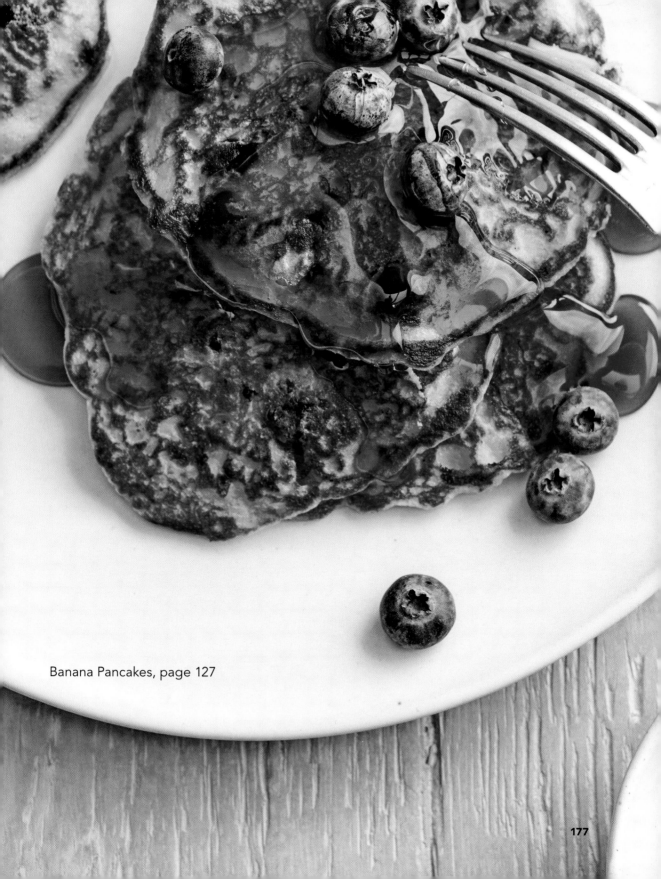

Banana Pancakes, page 127

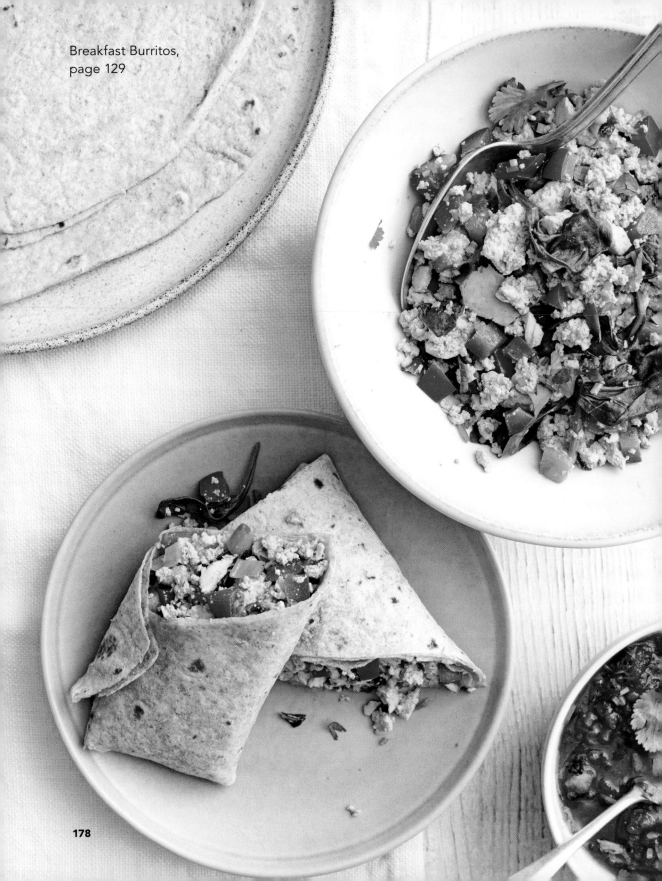

Breakfast Burritos,
page 129

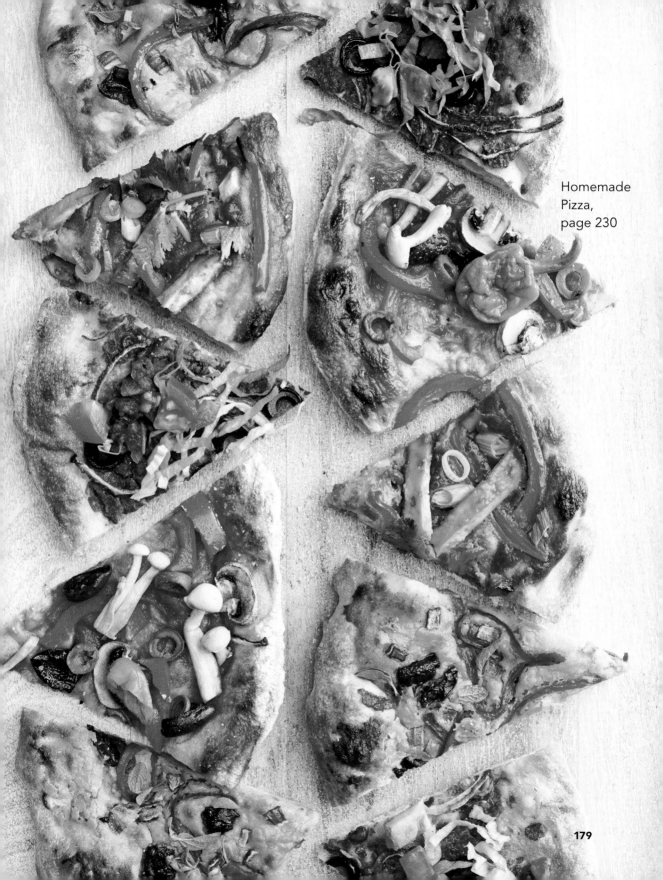

Homemade
Pizza,
page 230

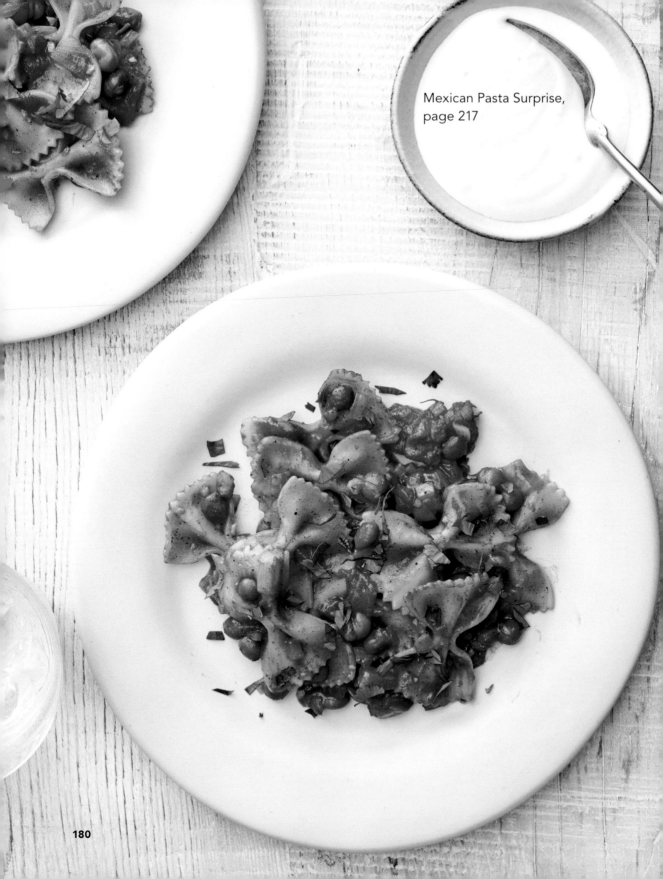

Mexican Pasta Surprise,
page 217

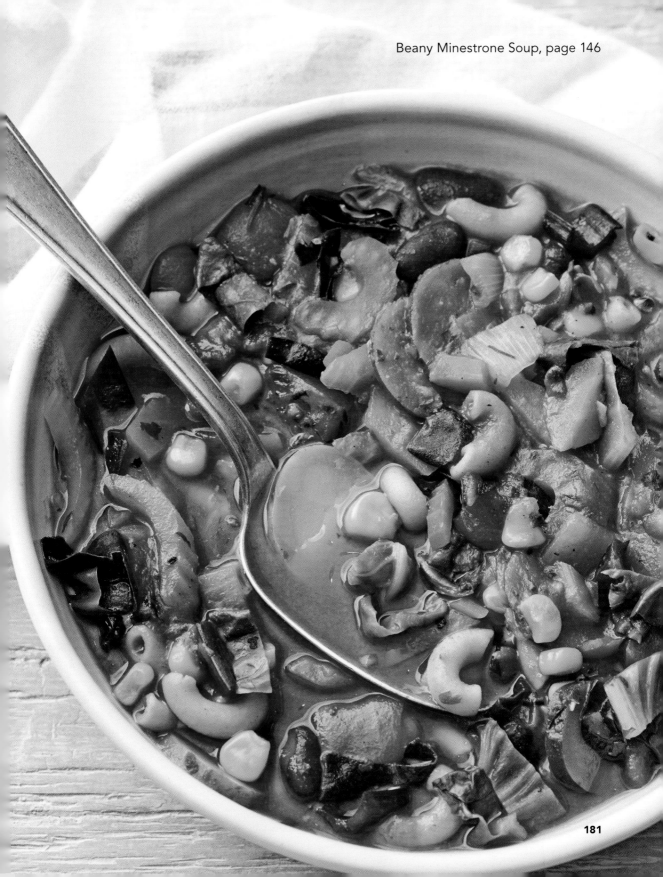

Beany Minestrone Soup, page 146

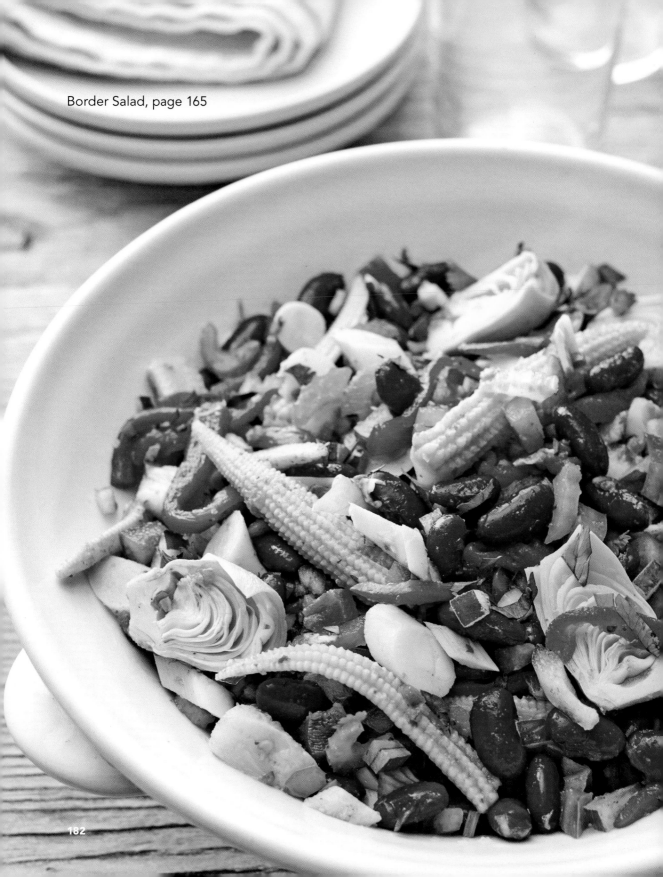

Border Salad, page 165

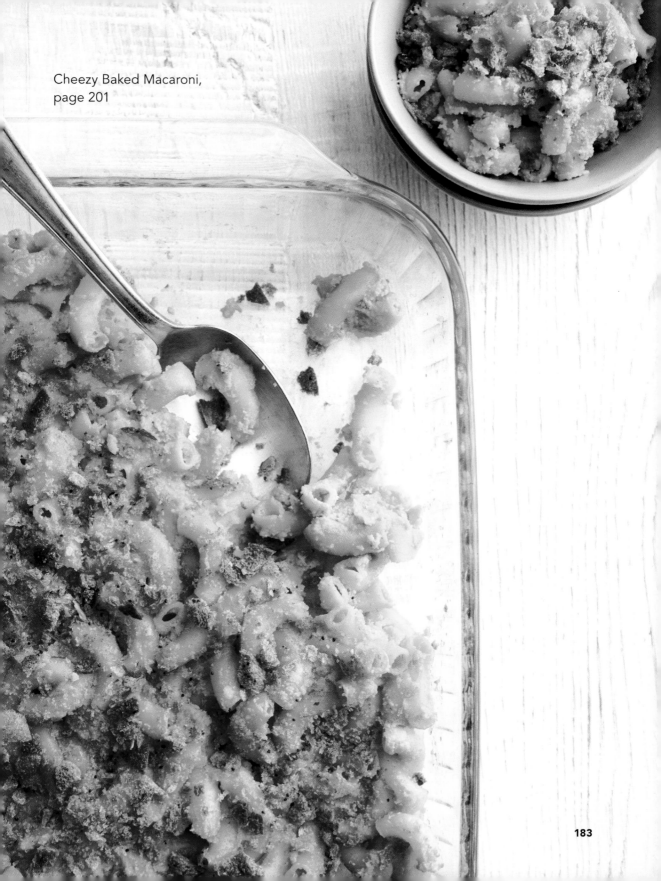

Cheezy Baked Macaroni,
page 201

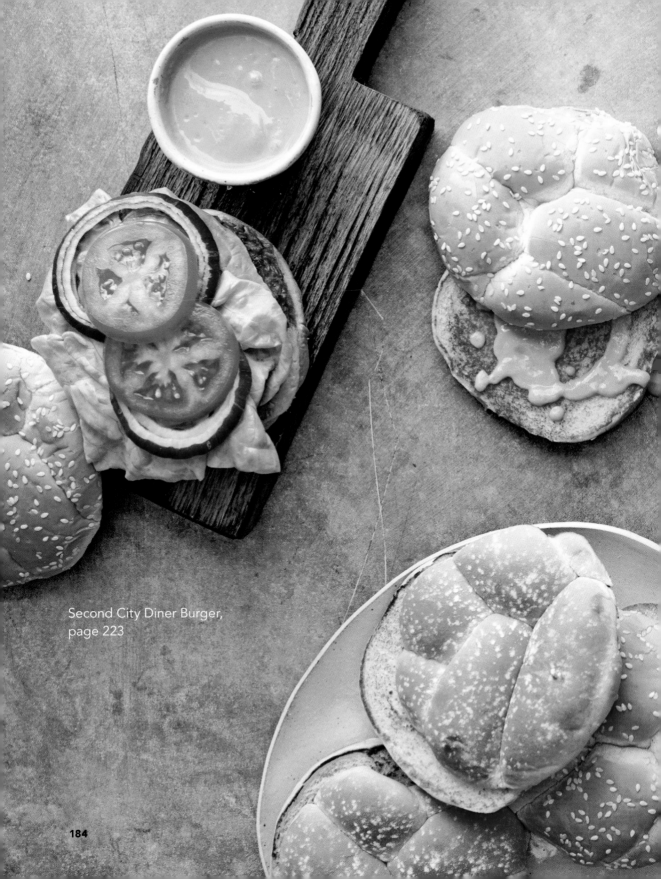

Second City Diner Burger,
page 223

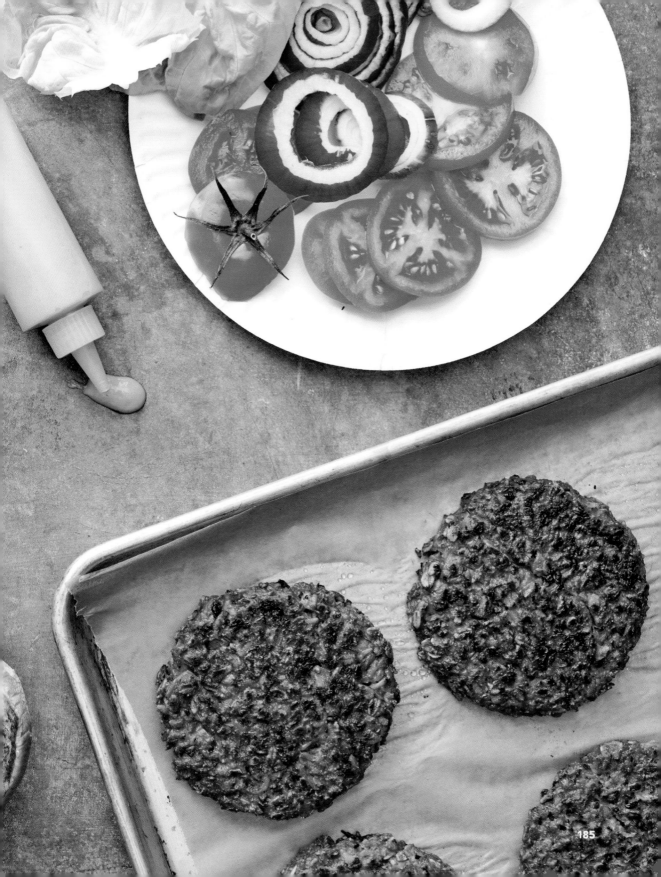

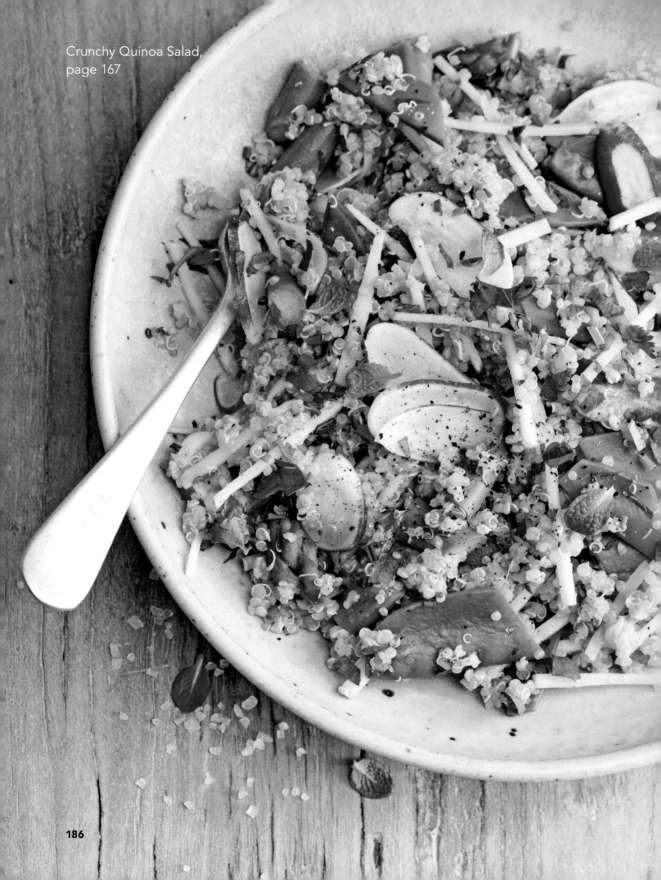

Crunchy Quinoa Salad,
page 167

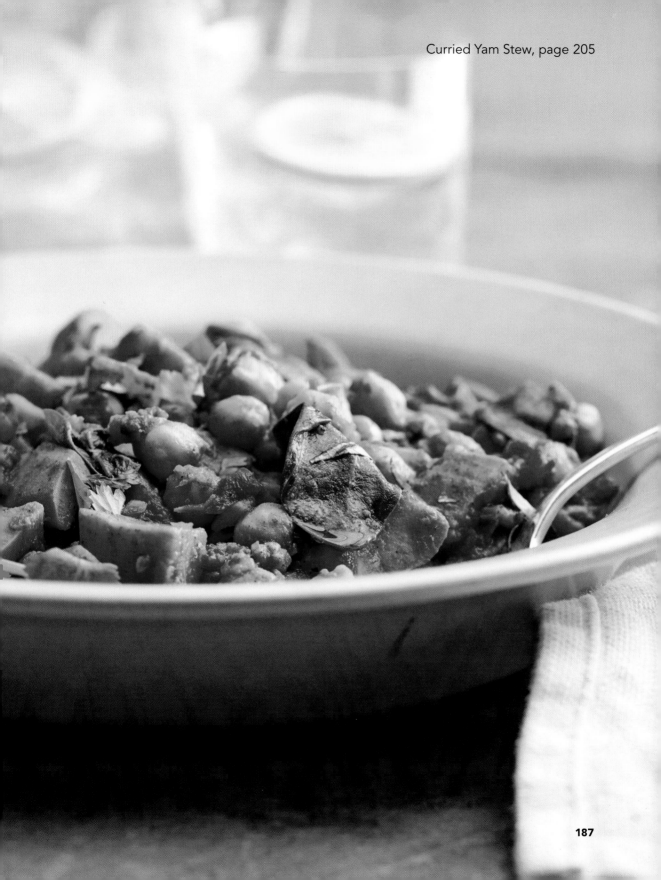

Curried Yam Stew, page 205

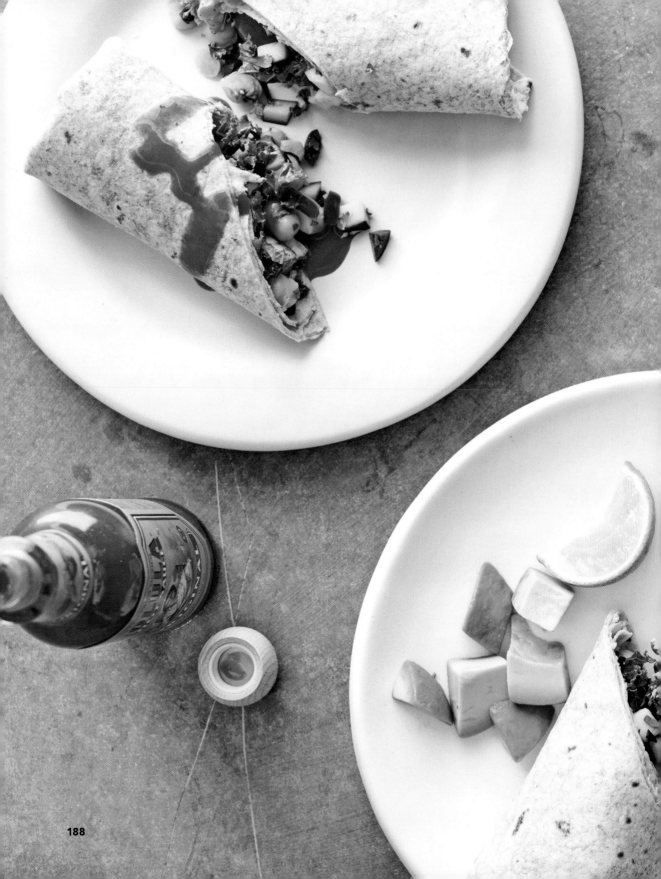

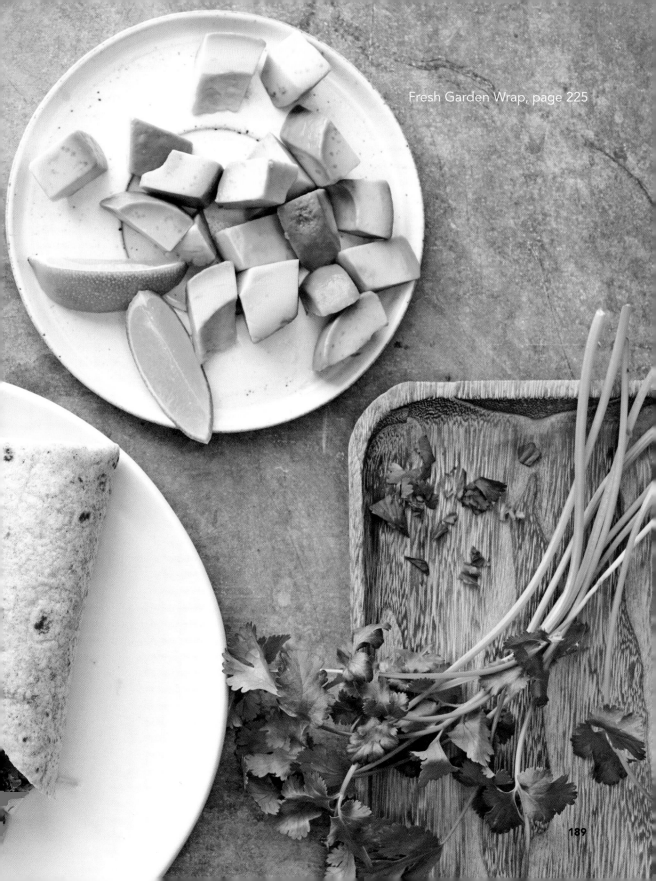

Fresh Garden Wrap, page 225

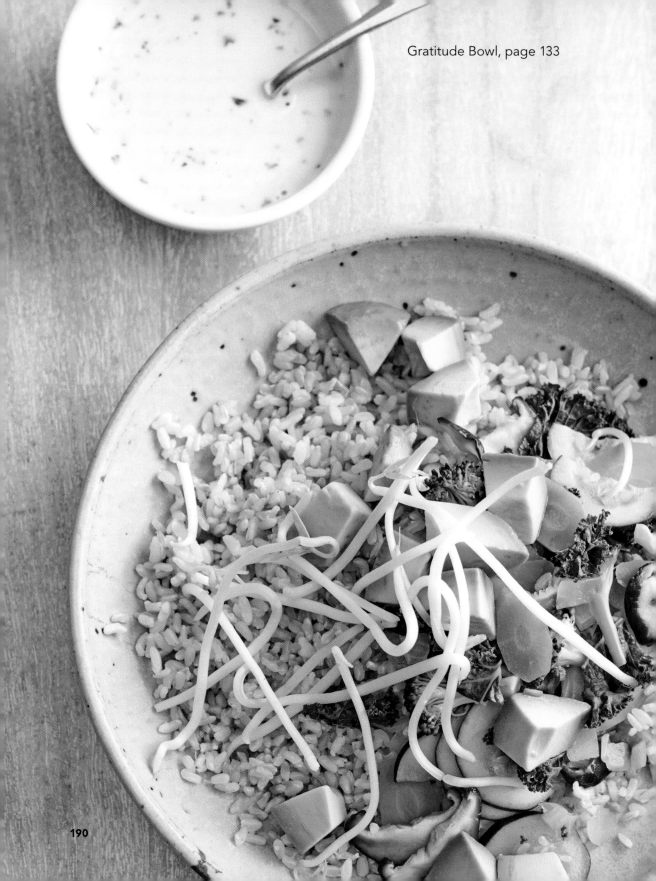

Gratitude Bowl, page 133

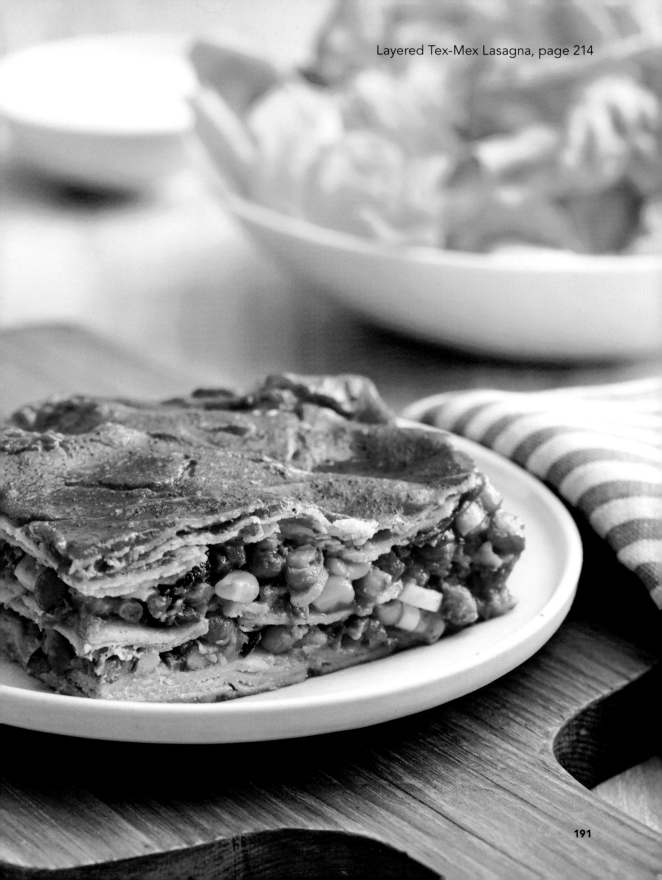

Layered Tex-Mex Lasagna, page 214

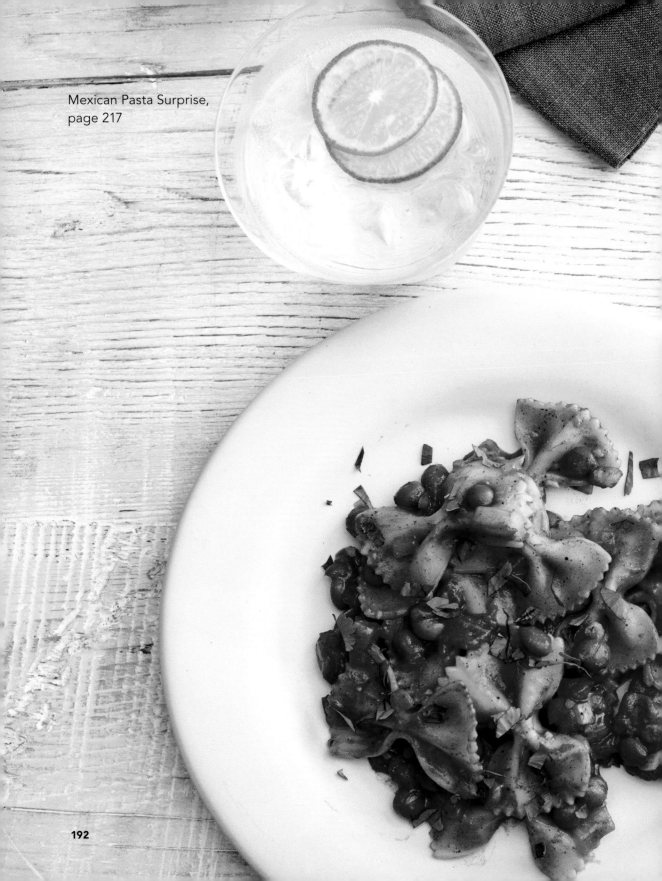

Mexican Pasta Surprise,
page 217

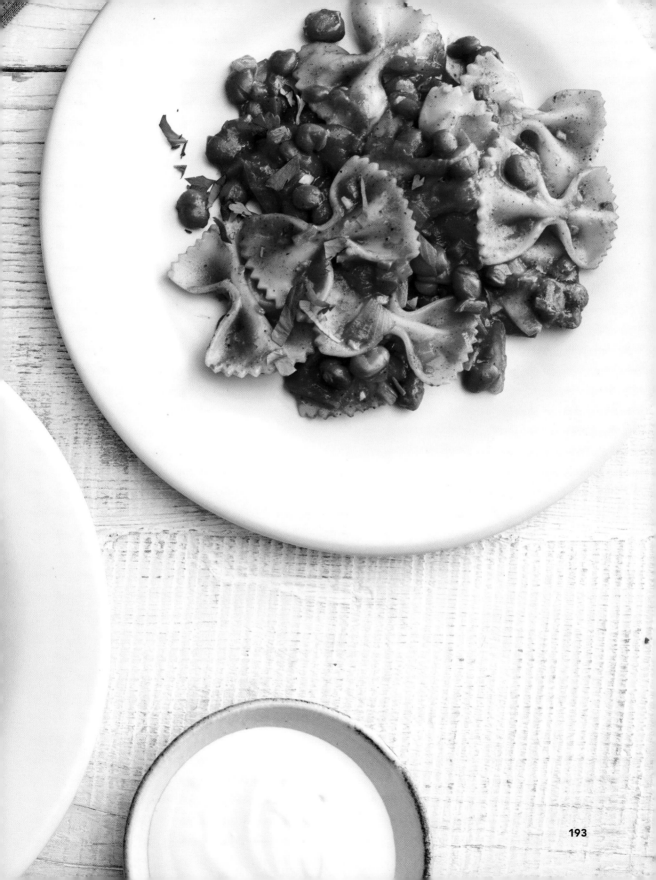

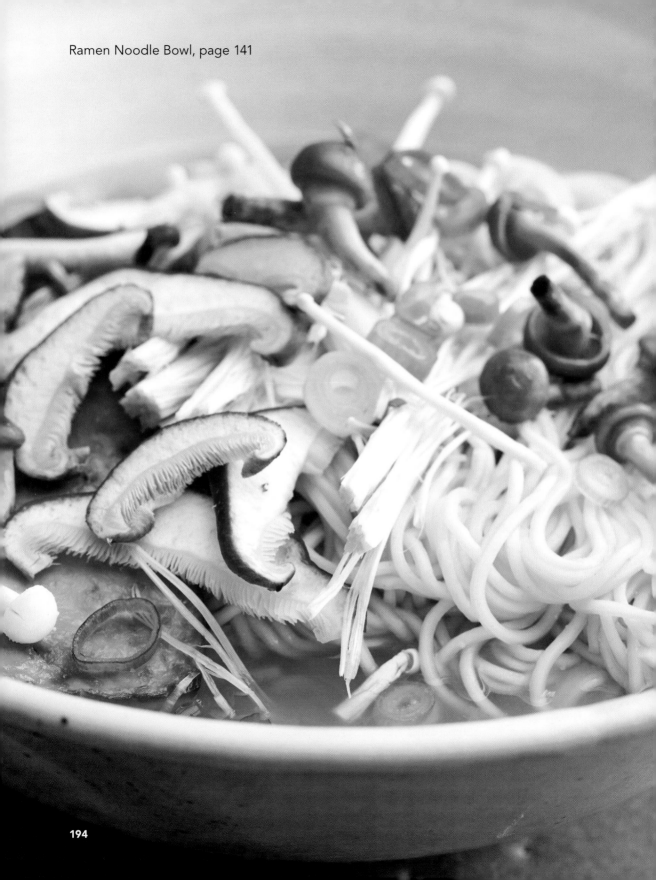

Ramen Noodle Bowl, page 141

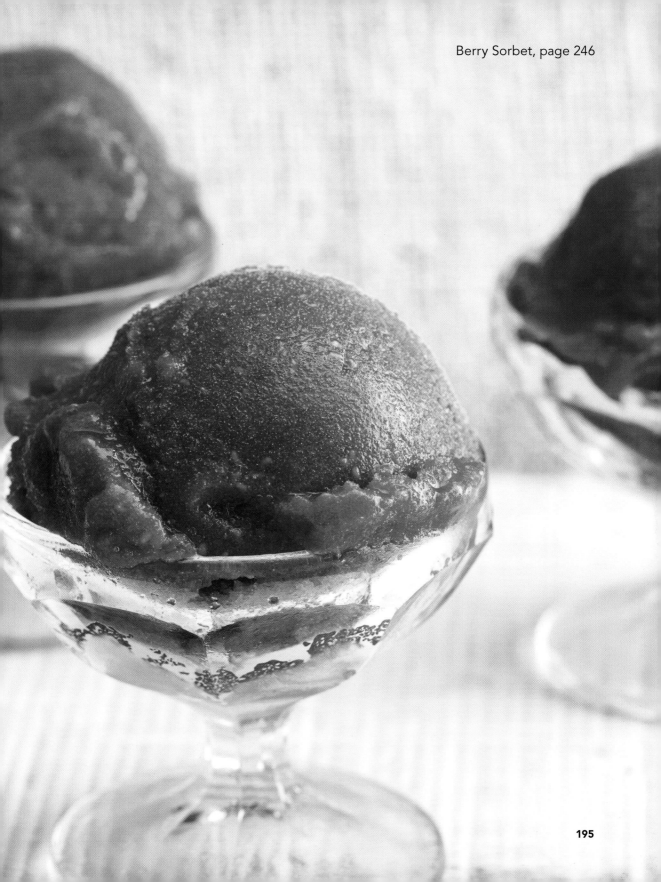

Berry Sorbet, page 246

Pear-Cranberry Crumble, page 247

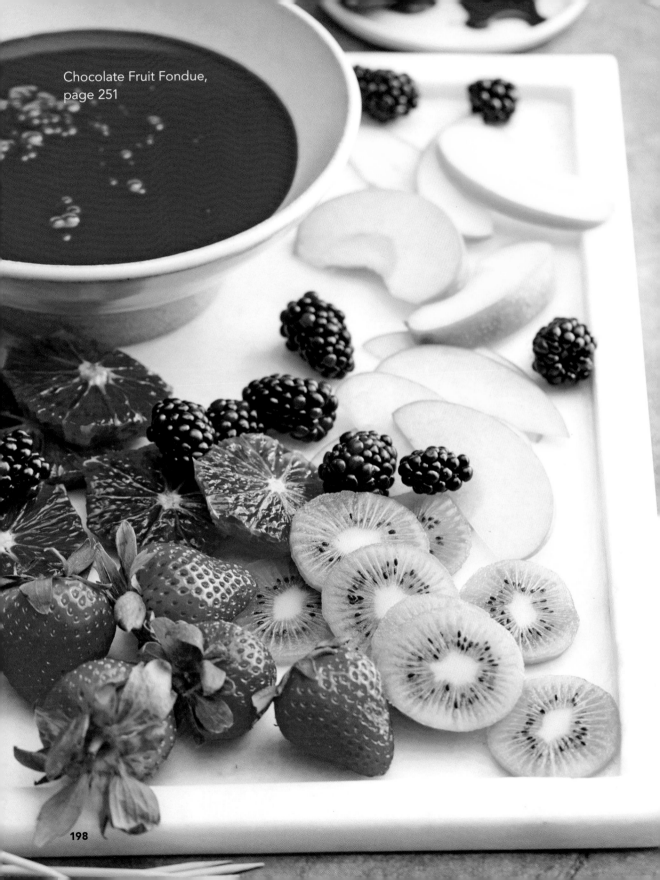

Chocolate Fruit Fondue,
page 251

Chana Masala

This is my very favorite curried garbanzo-bean dish. I always have canned garbanzo beans and tomatoes in my pantry and fresh spinach in my refrigerator, so I can prepare this easily whenever I get the urge.

Preparation Time: 20 minutes
Cooking Time: 40 minutes
Servings: 6 to 8

1 onion, chopped
2 cloves garlic, minced
1 teaspoon grated fresh ginger
2 tablespoons vegetable broth
1 tablespoon ground coriander
2 teaspoons ground cumin
1 teaspoon turmeric
½ teaspoon cayenne pepper
1 (14.5-ounce) can diced tomatoes
2 (15-ounce) cans garbanzo beans, drained and rinsed
1 (4-ounce) can chopped green chilies
1 cup water
4 cups coarsely chopped fresh spinach
2 to 3 tablespoons chopped fresh cilantro

Place the onion, garlic, and ginger in a large nonstick pot with the vegetable broth. Cook, stirring frequently, until onion softens slightly. Stir in the coriander, cumin, turmeric, and cayenne. Continue to cook and stir for 1 minute. Add the tomatoes and mix well. Then add the garbanzo beans, green chilies, and water. Bring to a boil, reduce the heat, cover, and cook for 20 minutes, adding a bit more water if it gets too thick. Add the spinach, mix well, and continue to cook for an additional 10 minutes. Sprinkle with the cilantro before serving.

Hint: To simplify this dish, substitute 2 tablespoons of curry powder for the coriander, cumin, turmeric, and cayenne.

Cheezy Baked Macaroni*

I have had many requests for a macaroni and cheese substitute, mainly from people with children. This recipe was developed with the children in mind, but I really like it too.

Preparation Time: 15 minutes
Cooking Time: 30 minutes
Servings: 6 to 8

---

12 ounces uncooked macaroni
1¼ cups raw cashews
1¼ cups water
¼ cup nutritional yeast
2½ tablespoons chopped pimientos
1 tablespoon lemon juice
2 teaspoons white miso
1 teaspoon onion powder
¼ teaspoon salt
¼ to ⅓ cup whole wheat bread crumbs

Preheat the oven to 350°F.

Place a large pot of water on to boil. Add the pasta to the boiling water and cook until just tender, about 6 minutes, depending on the kind of pasta used. Drain and set aside in a large bowl.

Meanwhile, place the cashews in a food processor with half of the water. Process until fairly smooth, then add the remaining ingredients, except the bread crumbs, and process for several minutes until the mixture is *very* smooth. Pour the mixture over the pasta and stir to combine. Transfer to a covered casserole dish, sprinkle the bread crumbs over the top, cover, and bake for 30 minutes.

Hints: Use any of your family's favorite tubular pasta in this recipe. The initial cooking time may have to be adjusted slightly depending on which type of pasta you choose. Cook until just tender; do not overcook, because the pasta will cook again while baking. This may be prepared ahead of time and refrigerated until ready to bake. Add about 10 minutes to the baking time.

Costa Rican Potatoes and Beans

We have been traveling to Costa Rica for many years and have enjoyed many delicious bean and rice dishes. I really enjoy this dish because of the potatoes!

Preparation Time: 30 minutes
Cooking Time: 30 minutes
Servings: 4

½ to 1 cup vegetable broth
1 onion, chopped
½ teaspoon minced fresh garlic
1 jalapeño pepper, seeded and minced
2½ cups chopped fresh tomatoes
¼ cup chopped fresh cilantro
Freshly ground black pepper
4 cups packed chopped spinach
3 cups chunked *cooked* potatoes
1 (15-ounce) can black beans, drained and rinsed
Hot sauce (optional)

Place ½ cup of the vegetable broth in a large nonstick frying pan. Add the onion, garlic, and jalapeño. Cook over medium heat, stirring frequently, until vegetables are very soft, adding the rest of the vegetable broth if necessary. Add tomatoes, cilantro, and black pepper. Cook, uncovered, over low heat, stirring occasionally, for 15 minutes.

Meanwhile, drop the spinach into boiling water for 1 minute. Drain and set aside. Add potatoes and beans to the tomato mixture. Mix well and cook for 3 minutes. Add spinach and cook for another minute. Season to taste with hot sauce. Serve hot or cold.

Curried Yam Stew*

This one-pot meal contains many of my favorite foods: garbanzo beans, spinach, and yams. It is easy to prepare, cooks quickly, and tastes delicious.

Preparation Time: 15 minutes
Cooking Time: 20 minutes
Servings: 4

4 cups peeled and diced garnet yams
1 (14.5-ounce) can diced tomatoes
1 (15-ounce) can garbanzo beans, drained and rinsed
¼ cup vegetable broth
2 teaspoons curry powder
½ teaspoon ground cumin
¼ teaspoon ground coriander
¼ teaspoon cinnamon
4 green onions, chopped
¼ cup chopped fresh cilantro
4 cups packed fresh baby spinach leaves

Place the yams, tomatoes, garbanzo beans, and broth in a large pot. Bring to a boil, reduce the heat, cover, and cook, stirring occasionally, for 15 minutes, until the yams are just tender. Add the remaining ingredients, except for the spinach leaves, and mix well. Place the spinach leaves on top of the stew, cover, and steam for 1 minute or so; then stir the leaves into the stew. Continue to cook, stirring frequently, for 4 minutes. Serve at once.

Easy Mayan Black Beans

This is one of those simple five-ingredient recipes that are so easy to put together, yet it has a delicious, hearty flavor. This will serve two people when used as a topping for baked potatoes or rolled up in a tortilla.

Preparation Time: 5 minutes
Cooking Time: 15 minutes
Servings: 2

1 (15-ounce) can black beans, drained and rinsed
1 cup fresh salsa (mild, medium, or hot)
½ cup chopped green onions
¾ cup frozen corn kernels
¼ cup chopped fresh cilantro (optional)

Place all the ingredients except the cilantro in a saucepan and bring to a gentle boil. Reduce the heat, cover, and cook for about 12 minutes, stirring occasionally. Stir in the cilantro, if desired. Let rest for 1 minute and serve.

Hints: This also makes a wonderful topping for brown rice. Or for a simple recipe variation, add about ¾ cup of cooked brown rice to the bean mixture about 5 minutes before the end of the cooking time. This recipe adapts well to precooking: double the recipe, cook ahead of time, refrigerate half for use within the next 2 days, and freeze the remainder for later use.

Farmhouse Bread Stew

The addition of bread to the stew during the last 5 minutes of cooking really makes this dish a special treat. This is a very hearty stew, best served in a wide, deep bowl.

Preparation Time: 15 minutes
Cooking Time: 1 hour, 10 minutes
Servings: 4

6 cups vegetable broth
1 onion, chopped
2 cloves garlic, minced
2 stalks celery, chopped
1 carrot, chopped
1 (14.5-ounce) can diced tomatoes
2 (15-ounce) cans red beans, drained and rinsed
¼ cup pearled barley
1 bay leaf
1 teaspoon dried oregano
Freshly ground black pepper to taste
3 cups chopped fresh spinach
2 cups cubed hearty bread

Place a small amount of the broth in a large soup pot. Add the onion, garlic, celery, and carrot. Cook, stirring occasionally, for about 5 minutes, until vegetable soften slightly. Add the remaining broth, canned tomatoes, beans, barley, bay leaf, oregano, and ground pepper. Bring to a boil, reduce the heat, cover, and cook for about 55 minutes. Add the spinach and cook for an additional

5 minutes. Then add the bread and cook for about 5 minutes longer. Serve at once.

Hints: If you prepare this stew ahead of time, do not add the bread until just before serving. A hearty artisan-type bread that is about 2 days old works very well in this recipe. Softer breads do not hold their shape well. I use small red beans in this recipe, but this could also be made with other kinds of beans, such as white or black.

Garden Potato Medley

We grew potatoes in our garden this year, and there is nothing better tasting than freshly dug potatoes. We also had a huge crop of heirloom tomatoes and plenty of dinosaur kale (my favorite variety), so this dish is a staple during the fall months.

Preparation Time: 15 minutes
Cooking Time: 20 minutes
Servings: 4

4 cups chunked potatoes
1 tablespoon vegetable broth
1 onion, chopped
1 teaspoon minced fresh garlic
1 jalapeño pepper, seeded and minced
2½ cups chopped fresh tomatoes
Freshly ground black pepper
4 cups packed chopped dinosaur kale
1 (15-ounce) can red beans, drained and rinsed
1 tablespoon low-sodium soy sauce
1 teaspoon chili paste (*sambal oelek*)
¼ cup chopped fresh cilantro

Place the potatoes in water to cover, bring to a boil, reduce the heat, and cook until fairly tender, 6 to 8 minutes. Drain and set aside.

Place the vegetable broth in a large nonstick frying pan. Add the onion, garlic, and jalapeño. Cook over medium heat, stirring frequently, until vegetables are very soft, 3 to 4 minutes. Add tomatoes and black pepper. Cook, uncovered, over low heat, stirring occasionally, for 3 minutes. Add the kale and stir gently to combine. Cover and continue to cook for about 2 minutes, until kale turns bright green; then add the potatoes and beans. Cook, stirring occasionally for 5 minutes; then add the soy sauce, chili paste, and cilantro. Cook an additional 5 minutes, until kale is tender. Serve warm or cold.

Hints: Use a variety of tomatoes for an attractive, colorful dish. Use small, new potatoes cooked with the skins on for best flavor. Small red potatoes or fingerlings are delicious in this recipe. If you can't get dinosaur kale (also called lacinato kale), use regular kale, but remove the stems first.

International Stew

I have prepared this stew several times during the past few weeks using different grains, making this dish truly international. I never have enough left over to freeze, but if you do, it may be frozen for later use. We like this by itself over brown rice in a bowl or scooped up with baked tortilla chips.

Preparation Time: 25 minutes
Cooking Time: 60 minutes
Servings: 6

---

3 cups vegetable broth
1 onion, chopped
2 stalks celery, chopped
2 carrots, chopped
1 green bell pepper, chopped
1 red bell pepper, chopped
3 cloves garlic, minced
2 cups baby potatoes, chunked
2 (15-ounce) cans white cannellini beans, drained and rinsed
1 (8-ounce) can tomato sauce
1½ cups prepared hummus
1½ tablespoons dried parsley flakes
1½ tablespoons low-sodium soy sauce
1 teaspoon dried basil
½ teaspoon dried oregano
½ teaspoon smoked paprika
⅛ to ¼ teaspoon crushed red pepper flakes
½ cup *cooked* quinoa
1½ cups thinly sliced fresh spinach

Place ½ cup of the broth in a large pot. Add onion, celery, carrot, bell pepper, and garlic. Cook, stirring occasionally, for 10 minutes. Add the remaining broth, potatoes, and beans. Bring to a boil, cover, reduce the heat, and cook for 30 minutes. Add the tomato sauce, hummus, and seasonings. Cook an additional 10 minutes. Add the cooked quinoa, mix well, and cook for 5 minutes. Stir in the spinach and cook an additional 2 minutes.

Hints: This may be made with other cooked grains, such as bulgur, kasha, millet, rice, or even whole wheat couscous (which is not a grain, but a pasta). Most natural-food stores sell prepared low-fat hummus, or you can easily make your own by pureeing cooked garbanzo beans with a small amount of broth, garlic, and salt. This stew may also be made with garbanzo beans instead of white beans. If you can't find baby potatoes, use larger red potatoes and cut them into bite-sized chunks. If you want to use chard or kale instead of spinach, cook it 5 additional minutes.

Harlequin Rice

Preparation Time: 15 minutes
Cooking Time: 50 minutes
Servings: 4

2¼ cups vegetable broth
1 onion, chopped
1 red bell pepper, chopped
½ cup chopped green onion
1 teaspoon minced fresh garlic
1 cup uncooked brown basmati rice
1 (4-ounce) can chopped green chilies
1 (4-ounce) jar chopped pimientos
1 cup fresh or frozen corn kernels
1 tablespoon dried parsley flakes
1 teaspoon ground cumin
2 cups packed chopped spinach
¼ cup chopped fresh cilantro
Freshly ground black pepper to taste

Place ¼ cup of the vegetable broth in a large pot with the onion, bell pepper, green onion, and garlic. Cook, stirring occasionally, until vegetables soften slightly, about 3 minutes. Add the remaining broth, the rice, green chilies, pimientos, corn, parsley, and cumin. Cover, bring to a boil, reduce the heat, and simmer for about 45 minutes, until rice is tender. Stir in the remaining ingredients and cook for 2 minutes longer.

Layered Tex-Mex Lasagna*

Preparation Time: 40 minutes
Cooking Time: 45 minutes
Servings: 6 to 8

12 corn tortillas
4 cups of cooked mashed pinto beans
1 cup chopped green onions
1½ cups frozen corn kernels, thawed
1 (2.25-ounce) can sliced ripe olives, drained
1 to 2 tablespoons chopped green chilies (optional)
Salsa (optional)
Tofu sour cream (optional; recipe available at
    www.drmcdougall.com)

SAUCE

2 (8-ounce) cans tomato sauce
3 cups water
4 tablespoons cornstarch
3 tablespoons chili powder
½ teaspoon onion powder
¼ teaspoon garlic powder

Place the beans in a large bowl. Add the onions, corn, olives, and green chilies (if using). Mix gently until well combined. Set aside.

For the sauce, place all the ingredients in a saucepan. Whisk until well combined. Cook and stir over medium heat until thickened, about 5 minutes. Taste and add more chili powder, if desired. Set aside.

Preheat the oven to 350°F.

Place 1½ cups of the sauce in the bottom of a nonstick 9 × 13-inch baking dish. Place 4 corn tortillas over the bottom of the baking dish; they can overlap or be cut to fit. Spread half of the bean mixture over the tortillas. Place another 4 tortillas over the bean mixture and then spread the remaining bean mixture on top of those tortillas. Cover with 4 more tortillas and then pour the remaining sauce over the tortillas. Cover with parchment paper and then with aluminum foil, crimping the edges over the baking dish. Bake for 45 minutes. Remove from the oven and let rest for about 15 minutes before cutting. Serve with salsa and tofu sour cream, if desired.

Mediterranean Garbanzo Beans

I developed this recipe on the same day that I made the Cheezy Baked Macaroni, thinking that our grandson Jaysen would love the pasta and that this dish would be too spicy for him. Well, he proved me wrong—he ate six bowls of this dish and only a few bites of the pasta! So I just never know which foods will appeal to which people, since we all have different tastes.

Preparation Time: 15 minutes
Cooking Time: 40 minutes
Servings: 6 to 8

2 onions, chopped
3 cloves garlic, minced
¼ cup vegetable broth
2 (15-ounce) cans garbanzo beans, drained and rinsed
1 (28-ounce) can crushed tomatoes with basil
1 large fresh tomato, chopped
1 teaspoon dried oregano
1 teaspoon crushed red pepper flakes
2 tablespoons lemon juice
4 cups packed chopped fresh spinach
Freshly ground black pepper

Place the onion and garlic in a large pot with the vegetable broth. Cook, stirring occasionally, until onion is tender, about 4 minutes. Add beans, tomatoes, oregano, and red pepper flakes. Mix well, bring to a boil, reduce the heat, cover, and cook for 30 minutes, stirring occasionally. Add the lemon juice, spinach, and several twists of freshly ground black pepper. Cook for an additional 5 minutes, until spinach is tender.

Mexican Pasta Surprise*

We don't very often think of pasta as part of a Mexican meal, but this combination of beans, pasta, and sauce has a wonderful flavor. It is also very quick to make, and almost everyone loves it. Choose a different shape pasta for variety.

Preparation Time: 20 minutes
Cooking Time: 45 minutes
Servings: 6

    8 ounces uncooked bow-tie pasta
    ¼ cup vegetable broth
    1 onion, chopped
    2 jalapeño peppers, seeded and minced
    1½ teaspoons minced fresh garlic
    ½ teaspoon chipotle chili powder
    1 (14.5-ounce) can stewed tomatoes
    1 (15-ounce) can pinto beans, drained and rinsed
    1¼ cups Enchilada Sauce
    ¼ cup chopped fresh cilantro (optional)
    ½ cup tofu sour cream (optional; recipe available at
        www.drmcdougall.com)

Place a large pot of water on to boil and cook pasta according to package directions. Drain and set aside.

Preheat the oven to 350°F.

Place the broth in a large nonstick pan. Add the onion, jalapeños, and garlic. Cook, stirring occasionally, until softened, about

5 minutes. Stir in the chipotle chili powder. Add the tomatoes, beans, and Enchilada Sauce (see the Sauces section). Mix well, breaking up the tomatoes slightly. Cook, stirring occasionally, for 10 minutes. Add the cooked pasta and mix well. Ladle the mixture into a casserole dish. Bake covered for 25 minutes. Uncover and bake for 5 minutes longer.

Serve with cilantro and tofu sour cream to spoon over each individual serving, if desired.

Hints: Cook the pasta until it is just tender; do not overcook. This dish may be prepared ahead of time and refrigerated until baking. You will need to add 10 to 15 minutes to the baking time. Chipotle chili powder is quite spicy. If you can't find it or would like a less spicy version, use regular chili powder instead.

Mushrooms, Kale, and Potatoes

Kale is a very nutritious vegetable, loaded with phytonutrients. This is delicious, healthy, and quick to put together. We like this with Sriracha hot sauce over the top for even more heat.

Preparation Time: 15 minutes
Cooking Time: 20 minutes
Servings: 2 to 3

3 cups red fingerling potatoes, chunked
2 onions, chopped
2 cloves garlic, minced
3 portobello mushrooms, coarsely chopped (see hints below)
6 cups packed coarsely chopped dinosaur kale
2 tablespoons low-sodium soy sauce
1 to 2 teaspoons chili paste (*sambal oelek*)
Freshly ground black pepper to taste

Place the potatoes in water to cover, bring to a boil, reduce the heat, and cook until fairly tender, 8 to 10 minutes. Drain and set aside.

Meanwhile, place the onion, garlic, and mushrooms in a large nonstick sauté pan or wok. Do not add any liquid. Dry-fry over medium heat, stirring frequently, for 5 to 6 minutes, until the onions and mushrooms are fairly tender. Add the kale and stir gently to combine. Continue to cook, stirring frequently, for about 2 minutes; then add the potatoes. Cook, stirring occasionally, for 5 minutes; then add the soy sauce, chili paste, and pepper. Cook an additional 5 minutes, until the kale is tender and the potatoes are somewhat browned. Serve warm.

Hints: Small red potatoes may be substituted for the fingerlings, if desired. If you can't get dinosaur kale (also called lacinato kale), use regular kale, but remove the stems first. I especially love this with about 4 cups of assorted, chopped exotic mushrooms, such as clamshell, trumpet royale, oyster, or chanterelle, in place of the portobellos. Many markets carry an assorted specialty mushroom package. Use about 1 pound total.

BURGERS, WRAPS, AND PIZZA

Grilled Portobello Burger

I like to make grilled portobello mushroom burgers for our family's Labor Day party. They are delicious, meaty, and easy to prepare on a gas or charcoal grill. Serve them on whole wheat buns with your favorite toppings. I like to have a variety of spreads to smear on the buns before adding lettuce, sliced tomatoes, and grilled onions.

Preparation Time: 10 minutes
Marinating Time: 30 minutes
Cooking Time: 10 minutes
Servings: 4

4 large portobello mushrooms
¼ cup low-sodium soy sauce
2 tablespoons rice vinegar
2 garlic cloves, crushed
1 teaspoon Dijon mustard
Freshly ground black pepper
4 thick slices red onion
Lettuce
Thickly sliced tomatoes
4 whole wheat burger buns
Assorted spreads (see hints below)

Clean the mushrooms well and remove the stems. Combine the soy sauce, vinegar, garlic, and Dijon mustard in a large bowl. Season with several twists of freshly ground black pepper. Add the mushrooms and onion slices, turning several times to coat them with the marinade. Let them soak in the marinade for about 30 minutes, turning several times. Remove the vegetables from the marinade, place them on a plate, and reserve the marinade for brushing.

Heat a gas grill to medium-high or light a charcoal grill. Grill the mushrooms and the onions for about 5 minutes on each side, brushing with extra marinade during grilling.

To serve, on the bun bottoms place a lettuce leaf, tomato slice, and grilled onion slice and top with the mushroom cap. Apply about 2 tablespoons of the spread of your choice to each of the bun tops and set on top of the mushrooms. Pick up with your hands and enjoy this delicious feast!

Hints: Some of our favorite spreads for these hearty burgers are Red Pepper Sauce, Tofu Chili Cream (see the Sauces section), tofu mayo, or some of the leftover Green Goddess sauce from the Green Goddess Potato Salad (see the Salads section). Or just keep it simple and use some ketchup and mustard.

Second City Diner Burger*

Vegetarian burgers made without soy, tofu, or beans are hard to find, so when I found this recipe online, I had to try it immediately. The recipe also included a very high-fat dressing to serve over the burger, which I modified into a much lower-fat version (see Red Pepper Sauce in the Sauces section). The sauce makes the burger very special, so give it a try! These were a hit with all of my family members, although some of them preferred the burger with more traditional burger toppings.

Preparation Time: 30 minutes
Chilling Time: 1 hour
Cooking Time: 45 minutes
Yield: 14 to 15 burgers

---

4 cups water
1 onion, finely chopped
3 stalks celery, finely chopped
¼ cup low-sodium soy sauce
2 teaspoons onion powder
2 teaspoons garlic powder
½ teaspoon freshly ground black pepper
3 cups rolled oats (not quick-cooking)
12 ounces mushrooms, finely chopped
½ cup white whole wheat flour

Place the water in a large pot with the onion, celery, soy sauce, onion powder, and garlic powder. Bring to a boil, reduce the heat, and simmer for 5 minutes. Stir in the oats, mushrooms, and flour and cook 5 minutes longer. Transfer to a bowl and chill for at least 1 hour, preferably longer.

Preheat the oven to 350°F.

Shape the mixture into burger-sized patties and place on the baking sheets. Bake for 15 minutes. Remove from the oven and let rest for 5 minutes (see hints below). Carefully flip over and bake 10 more minutes.

Before serving, place the baked patties on a nonstick griddle and grill for about 7 minutes on each side, until browned. Serve on buns with Red Pepper Sauce.

Hints: These burgers are quite fragile until after they are baked, so use extra care when flipping them for the first time. I found it works best if I let them rest out of the oven for at least 5 minutes before trying to loosen them from the pans. Use high-quality nonstick baking sheets for this recipe or line your baking sheets with silicone liners or parchment paper.

Fresh Garden Wrap*

This is another of our favorite summer meals, made with freshly harvested veggies from the garden.

Preparation Time: 15 minutes
Chilling Time: 1 hour
Servings: 6 to 8

---

 1 cup cherry tomatoes, cut in half
 1 cup shredded kale or bok choy
 1 zucchini, chopped
 1 cup broccoli florets
 ½ cup chopped green onions
 1 (15-ounce) can garbanzo beans, drained and rinsed
 1 tablespoon chopped Kalamata olives
 3 tablespoons red wine vinegar
 1 clove garlic, crushed
 1 tablespoon chopped fresh parsley
 ½ tablespoon chopped fresh cilantro
 6 to 8 whole wheat or corn tortillas
 Hot sauce (optional)

Place the vegetables and beans in a large bowl. Sprinkle the olives over the vegetables. Combine the vinegar, garlic, parsley, and cilantro in a small bowl. Pour over the vegetables and toss to mix. Cover and chill for at least 1 hour before serving.

To serve, place a line of the vegetable mixture down the center of a tortilla. Drizzle with hot sauce, if desired, roll up, and enjoy.

Hints: Try this with cucumber instead of zucchini. If you don't have kale or bok choy, use romaine lettuce instead. Use a few tablespoons of chopped avocado in place of the olives.

Mexican Picadillo Wraps

Wraps are a simple yet hearty meal for lunch or dinner. These are especially quick, because they make use of canned beans and leftover rice.

Preparation Time: 15 minutes
Cooking Time: 44 minutes
Servings: 8 to 10

½ cup water
1 onion, chopped
1 red bell pepper, chopped
1 teaspoon minced fresh garlic
2 (15-ounce) cans pinto beans, drained and rinsed
1 (14.5-ounce) can fire-roasted diced tomatoes
1 (4-ounce) can diced green chilies
1 tart green apple, cored and chopped
Freshly ground black pepper
2 cups *cooked* long-grain brown rice
½ cup raisins
1 (2.25-ounce) can sliced black olives, drained
¼ cup chopped fresh cilantro
2 tablespoons toasted slivered almonds (optional)
Corn or whole wheat tortillas
Hot sauce (optional)

Place the water in a large pot. Add the onion, bell pepper, and garlic. Cook, stirring occasionally, until the onion softens slightly, about 5 minutes. Add the beans, tomatoes, green chilies, apple, and several twists of freshly ground black pepper. Bring to a boil, reduce the heat, cover, and cook for 20 minutes on low. Add the remaining ingredients (except tortillas and hot sauce), mix well, and cook for 5 minutes until heated through.

Serve rolled up in tortillas with some hot sauce sprinkled over the top, if desired.

Hints: To toast the almonds, cook and stir in a dry nonstick pan until golden in color. This dish may also be made with black beans or 1 can of pinto and 1 can of black.

Specialdillas

These are delicious for either breakfast, lunch, or dinner! These can be served with salsa (and guacamole, if desired) spooned over the top and eaten with a knife and fork or cut into wedges, picked up with your fingers, and dunked into the salsa and/or guacamole.

Preparation Time: 20 minutes
Cooking Time: 5 minutes for each specialdilla
Servings: 8

2 pounds garnet yams, peeled and chunked
2 tablespoons vegetable broth
2 tablespoons chopped green chilies
2 teaspoons lime juice
1 teaspoon minced chipotle chilies in adobo sauce
¾ teaspoon ground cumin
½ teaspoon minced fresh garlic
1 (15-ounce) can black beans, drained and rinsed
8 whole wheat flour tortillas
Salsa
Guacamole (optional)

Peel the yams and place them in a stainless-steel saucepan with enough water to cover. Bring to a boil, reduce the heat, cover, and cook for about 12 minutes, until soft. Drain the water off and add the vegetable broth. Mash with a potato masher until quite smooth, then stir in the green chilies, lime juice, chipotle chilies, cumin, and garlic. Mix well; stir in the black beans and mix again.

Heat a nonstick griddle or large sauté pan over medium heat. Spread some of the yam mixture on one half of a tortilla, fold over, and flatten. Place the tortilla on the griddle and cook for about 2½ minutes on each side, flipping several times to make sure it doesn't burn. Repeat with the remaining ingredients. Serve with salsa and guacamole, if desired.

Hints: This recipe makes 8 specialdillas; however, they store well in the refrigerator and can be reheated on the griddle the next day to taste just like fresh-made.

Homemade Pizza*

Dough

I make a double batch of this dough and put it in the freezer. This way, I always have it on hand. You can make this dough into any size pizza you want.

Preparation Time: 10 minutes
Rising Time: 18 to 24 hours
Rolling Time: 30 minutes
Yield: 3 to 6 pizza crusts

---

 7 cups all-purpose or whole wheat flour (or a combination
   of the two)
 1 teaspoon active dry yeast
 1 to 2 teaspoons salt
 3 cups water, plus more if the dough is too dry

In a stand mixer with dough hook, add flour, yeast, and salt and mix on low speed until combined. Slowly add water until combined; then knead with the dough hook for 2 more minutes, or until dough starts to pull away from bowl and form a ball on hook. If the mixture seems too dry, add a bit more water. (Sometimes I need to do this, other times I do not. Not sure why.)

Put this mixture in a large clean bowl, cover with plastic wrap or silicone cover (I cover it with a towel too; not sure if that makes any difference, but it makes me feel better), and place in a draft-free area for 18 to 24 hours.

The next day, turn the mixture out onto a floured work surface. Shape into a long oval and cut it into 6 even sections, or 3 if you like your pizza thicker. Next, take a section and fold the ends toward the middle, flip it over, shape it into a ball, and place it on a baking sheet lined with parchment paper. Repeat with all sections. Cover the dough with plastic wrap and a towel and let sit for 1 hour. If you don't want to use the dough right away, simply place it in plastic bags and store it in the freezer.

After 1 hour, roll out each ball on a floured surface until it is the thickness you like your pizza. You can roll the dough out with a rolling pin or stretch it with your fingers. I like to place the rolled-out dough on a large wooden pizza spatula topped with parchment paper and a sprinkling of cornmeal, but a pan with a sprinkling of cornmeal will work too.

Toppings

Next, put the toppings on the crust. Some of our favorite pizzas are:

Mexican: refried beans, black olives, and onions; top with lettuce, tomatoes, and salsa after cooking

Thai: peanut sauce, red peppers, baked tofu, and onions; top with fresh cilantro and/or greens after cooking

Veggie: tomato sauce, red peppers, mushrooms, black and green olives, onions, and pepperoncinis

Greek: hummus, Kalamata olives, roasted red bell peppers, and red onions

Bake

I bake my pizza on a preheated pizza stone in my barbecue, on as high as it will go, for about 8 minutes. Alternately, you can bake the pizza on a pan in a 400°F oven for 10 to 15 minutes, depending on thickness.

Gluten-Free Dough

Yield: 3 medium pizzas (see hints below)

3 cups gluten-free flour (see hints below)
1 to 2 teaspoons salt
1 teaspoon yeast
1 tablespoon egg replacer mixed with 2 tablespoons warm water
1 teaspoon cider vinegar
1½ cups water

Mix dry ingredients in a stand mixer with a dough hook. Slowly add egg replacer mixture, vinegar, and water. Knead with the hook for 3 minutes. Then follow the regular dough instructions above.

Hints: You can easily double this gluten-free dough recipe. If you use Bob's Red Mill Gluten-Free Bread Mix for the gluten-free flour, omit the salt and use the yeast provided.

Asian Salad Dressing

Preparation Time: 3 minutes

Yield: 1 cup

⅓ cup water

¼ cup rice vinegar

¼ cup low-sodium soy sauce

½ teaspoon crushed red pepper flakes (optional)

¼ teaspoon minced fresh garlic

¼ teaspoon grated fresh ginger

¼ teaspoon guar gum

Combine all ingredients in a small jar with a lid and shake until well mixed.

Hint: Guar gum is a thickening agent that does not require cooking. It gives oil-free dressings a thicker consistency that clings well to salad leaves.

Asian Ginger Sauce

Preparation Time: 5 minutes
Cooking Time: 5 minutes
Yield: 1½ cups

¾ cup water
½ cup low-sodium soy sauce
¼ cup rice vinegar
1 tablespoon mirin
1 tablespoon agave nectar
1 teaspoon crushed fresh garlic
1 teaspoon grated fresh ginger
½ teaspoon crushed red pepper flakes
2 tablespoons cornstarch

Combine all ingredients in a saucepan and whisk until smooth. Bring to a boil while stirring and cook and stir until thickened. Serve warm over grains and vegetables.

Creamy Golden Gravy

This gravy is made with brown-rice flour instead of wheat flour. The great thing about using rice flour for thickening is that it doesn't form lumps as wheat flour often does. You can just sprinkle it over the top of a hot liquid, stir it in, and it thickens nicely; or mix it in before cooking and stir occasionally until thickened.

Preparation Time: 5 minutes
Cooking Time: 10 minutes
Yield: 2 cups

    2 cups vegetable broth
    3 tablespoons low-sodium soy sauce
    2 tablespoons tahini
    ¼ cup brown-rice flour
    Freshly ground black pepper
    Hot sauce, such as Sriracha (optional)

Place the broth in a saucepan. Add the soy sauce and tahini. Stir in the brown-rice flour and whisk until the liquid becomes smooth. Bring to a boil, stirring occasionally, until the sauce becomes thickened. Season with freshly ground black pepper to taste. Add a dash or two of hot sauce for more flavor, if desired. Serve at once.

Hints: This gravy may be made ahead and refrigerated. It will thicken slightly when refrigerated. To reheat, place the gravy in a saucepan, add a small amount of water, and whisk to combine; then heat slowly, stirring occasionally, until hot.

Enchilada Sauce

Preparation Time: 5 minutes
Cooking Time: 5 minutes
Yield: 2½ cups

1 (8-ounce) can tomato sauce
1½ cups water
2 tablespoons cornstarch
1½ tablespoons chili powder
¼ teaspoon chipotle chili powder
¼ teaspoon onion powder
⅛ teaspoon garlic powder

Combine all ingredients in a saucepan and whisk until smooth. Cook and stir over medium heat until thickened.

Marinara Sauce

This is my family's favorite simple marinara sauce, which I have been making the same way for over thirty years.

Preparation Time: 20 minutes
Cooking Time: 1 hour, 10 minutes
Yield: about 4 cups

2 tablespoons water
2 onions, chopped
4 cloves garlic, crushed
½ pound mushrooms, chopped
2 (15-ounce) cans tomato sauce
1 (14.5-ounce) can diced tomatoes
1½ tablespoons dried parsley flakes
2 teaspoons dried oregano
1 teaspoon dried basil
Dash sea salt (optional)

Place the water, onions, garlic, and mushrooms in a large pot. Cook, stirring frequently, until the onions soften and begin to take on a golden color, about 10 minutes. Stir in the remaining ingredients. Bring to a boil, reduce the heat, and simmer for about 1 hour, stirring occasionally. Do not cover. Serve over pasta.

Hints: This may be made ahead and reheated. It also freezes well.

Mushroom-Tomato Sauce

This is a delicious tomato sauce that is wonderful on pasta, baked potatoes, or rice. It tastes even better the day after it is made and may also be frozen.

Preparation Time: 20 minutes
Cooking Time: 1 hour
Yield: about 7 cups

4 cups water, *divided*
2 onions, chopped
2 to 3 cloves garlic, minced
1 (28-ounce) can tomato puree
Freshly ground black pepper
1 pound portobello mushrooms, chopped
½ pound cremini mushrooms, sliced
¼ to ⅓ cup chopped fresh basil

Place ½ cup of water in a large pot. Add 1 cup of the chopped onions and 1 teaspoon of the minced garlic. Cook, stirring frequently, until the onion and garlic soften slightly, about 5 minutes. Add the tomato puree and 3 cups of water. Season with several twists of freshly ground black pepper. Bring to a boil, reduce the heat to low, and simmer for about 30 minutes, stirring occasionally.

Meanwhile, place the remaining ½ cup of water in a large nonstick frying pan. Add the remaining onions and garlic and cook, stirring frequently, until the onions and garlic soften slightly. Add all the mushrooms and continue to cook, stirring occasionally, until the mushrooms are tender, about 5 minutes. Add to the tomato mixture and cook over low heat for about 30 minutes longer, stirring occasionally. Remove from the heat and stir in the basil. Season with more freshly ground black pepper and a bit of salt, if desired.

Peanut-Hoisin Sauce

This is a higher-fat choice because of the peanut butter. Use over grain or noodle dishes or as a topping for potatoes or vegetables.

Preparation Time: 10 minutes
Yield: 1 cup

½ cup natural chunky peanut butter (no salt, sugar, or added oil)
½ cup water
2 tablespoons hoisin sauce
1 tablespoon low-sodium soy sauce
½ tablespoon agave nectar
2 teaspoons chili-garlic sauce
2 teaspoons tomato paste
1 teaspoon lime juice
½ teaspoon grated fresh ginger
Dash sesame oil (optional)

Place all ingredients in a food processor and process briefly until well combined but not smooth. Pour into a covered container and refrigerate until ready to use. Sauce may be heated before serving, if desired.

Red Pepper Sauce

Use this as a dip for raw veggies or crackers or as a spread on bread or veggie burger buns.

Preparation Time: 10 minutes
Chilling Time: 1 hour or longer
Yield: 2 cups

---

1 (12.3-ounce) package soft silken tofu
2 tablespoons lemon juice
1 tablespoon apple cider vinegar
Dash salt
½ cup roasted red bell peppers (see hint below)

Place the tofu in a food processor and process until fairly smooth. Add the remaining ingredients and process until very smooth (this may take several minutes). Refrigerate at least 1 hour to blend flavors.

Hint: You may either buy jarred roasted red bell peppers (just be sure they are not packed in oil) or roast your own.

Szechuan Sauce

Preparation Time: 10 minutes
Cooking Time: 5 minutes
Yield: 1½ cups

1½ cups water
5 to 6 green onions, chopped
2 tablespoons low-sodium soy sauce
1½ tablespoons cornstarch
¾ tablespoon minced fresh ginger
1 clove garlic, crushed
⅛ teaspoon crushed red pepper flakes
Dash hot sauce, such as Sriracha

Combine all ingredients in a saucepan and mix well. Cook and stir over medium heat until the mixture is thickened and clear, about 5 minutes.

Tahini Lemon Sauce

This is a higher-fat sauce because of the tahini, which is made from sesame seeds. Use only a small amount to season your bowl, or choose one of the nonfat sauces from this book for a lower-fat option.

Preparation Time: 5 minutes
Yield: 2 cups

1 cup water
¾ cup tahini
⅓ cup lemon juice
2 cloves garlic, minced
½ tablespoon low-sodium soy sauce
¼ teaspoon crushed red pepper flakes

Place all ingredients in a blender and process until smooth. Refrigerate in a covered container for up to 1 week.

Thai Peanut Sauce

Although most Thai peanut sauces use coconut milk in their preparation, I have used almond milk with coconut extract instead to reduce the fat. However, this sauce does contain some fat from the peanut butter.

Preparation Time: 5 minutes
Cooking Time: 5 minutes
Yield: ¾ cup

½ cup almond milk
¼ cup natural peanut butter (no salt, sugar, or added oil)
1 tablespoon low-sodium soy sauce
½ tablespoon agave nectar
1 teaspoon lime juice
1 teaspoon chili-garlic sauce
⅛ teaspoon coconut extract
1 to 2 tablespoons chopped fresh cilantro (optional)

Place all ingredients in a blender or food processor and process until smooth. Pour into a saucepan and heat through before serving. Serve warm over grains and vegetables.

Tofu Chili Cream

This cream is delicious and easy to make, and is wonderful stirred into Creamy Corn Soup for a bit more heat, or try it on top of burritos, tacos, or wraps.

Preparation Time: 5 minutes
Yield: about 1 cup

6 to 8 ounces silken tofu
2 to 4 tablespoons canned chopped green chilies
1 teaspoon minced fresh garlic

Place all ingredients in a blender jar and process until smooth. Scrape the sides as necessary and repeat until well processed. Place in a bowl and chill until served.

Hint: Make this sauce 1 to 2 days ahead of time to allow the flavors to blend.

DESSERTS

Berry Sorbet*

Preparation Time: 10 minutes
Chilling Time: 6 to 8 hours
Servings: 8

---

4 cups frozen raspberries or strawberries
1½ cups water
½ cup agave nectar
2 tablespoons lemon juice

Place the frozen berries in a bowl on the counter and allow to partially thaw. Do not drain.

Place the berries in a blender or food processor and process until smooth. Add the remaining ingredients and process again. Pour into a bowl. Cover and freeze until slushy, about 3 hours. Beat with an electric mixer until smooth. Cover and return to freezer. Freeze until firm, several more hours or overnight.

Remove from freezer about 10 minutes before serving.

Hints: To make this with sugar instead of agave, use about 1 cup of sugar dissolved in 1½ cups of boiling water in a saucepan. Remove from the heat and cool completely. Try this with fresh melon of any kind instead of berries. Use about ½ cup of orange juice instead of the lemon juice.

Pear-Cranberry Crumble*

I had some fresh cranberries in my refrigerator that our grandson Jaysen wanted to use. I also had fresh pears, so we decided to make a dessert. While it was cooling on the rack, everyone came in for a sample, and we all decided it was a hit!

Preparation Time: 20 minutes
Cooking Time: 1 hour
Servings: 8 to 10

TOPPING

½ cup rolled oats
½ cup chopped walnuts
¼ cup white whole wheat flour
½ teaspoon cinnamon
¼ teaspoon ground nutmeg
2 tablespoons agave nectar

FILLING

3 cups peeled, cubed Bosc pears
2 cups fresh cranberries
⅓ cup brown sugar
2½ tablespoons cornstarch

Preheat the oven to 350°F.

Combine the dry topping ingredients in a medium bowl and mix well; then add the agave and mix again until crumbly. Set aside.

Place pears, cranberries, brown sugar, and cornstarch in a large bowl. Mix until well combined. Transfer to a deep-dish pie plate and sprinkle the topping mixture over the top. Bake for about 1 hour, until the filling is bubbly and the top is slightly browned. Cool for 1 hour (if you can wait!).

Hints: I used Bosc pears because they tend to keep their shape when cooked and don't get too mushy. When fresh cranberries are not available, frozen (thawed) berries may be used in their place. My family likes this plain, but for a special treat you may want to top this with some rice or soy vanilla "ice cream."

Frozen Banana Dessert

This is just like soft-serve ice cream. You must use a food processor, not a blender, for this recipe. Depending on the size of your food processor, you may have to make this in 2 batches.

Preparation Time: 5 minutes
Servings: 6

---

5 to 6 very ripe, peeled *frozen* bananas (frozen overnight or longer)
1 tablespoon vanilla
½ cup nondairy milk

Break frozen bananas into 1-inch pieces. Place them in a food processor with the vanilla and nondairy milk and puree until creamy, stopping the machine occasionally to stir so that it processes evenly. Serve immediately. This may also be refrozen, if you do not want to eat all of it at one time. Thaw slightly before serving after freezing.

Hint: Frozen mangoes, strawberries, raspberries, or other fruit of choice may be substituted for up to a third of the bananas.

Banana-Strawberry Delight

This is a delicious, thick pudding-like dessert that is even better made with fresh strawberries when they are available. Use about 2 cups of fresh sliced strawberries in place of the frozen ones.

Preparation Time: 30 minutes
Cooking Time: 20 minutes
Chilling Time: 2 hours
Servings: 8

4 ripe bananas, cut up
1½ tablespoons lemon juice
1 (16-ounce) package of frozen, unsweetened strawberries, thawed
2 cups water
½ cup quick-cooking tapioca

Place the bananas and lemon juice in a blender jar and blend until smooth. Place the banana mixture in a saucepan. Add the thawed strawberries and their juice. Add the water and tapioca. Mix well. Let stand 5 minutes. Heat to boiling, stirring frequently. Remove from the heat. Let stand for 20 minutes. Then stir and spoon into dessert cups. Refrigerate until chilled, about 2 hours.

Hints: Try frozen raspberries instead of strawberries. While mixture is cooking, gently crush berries against side of pan to release more flavor and color.

Chocolate Fruit Fondue*

This dessert is a big favorite with children and adults alike. I have an old fondue pot from the 1970s that I still use to heat the chocolate sauce and keep it warm. To serve more people, just double the sauce amounts.

Preparation Time: 5 to 10 minutes
Cooking Time: 10 minutes
Yield: 1 cup sauce (serves 2 with fruit)

1 tablespoon Wonderslim Wondercocoa powder
2 teaspoons cornstarch or arrowroot
2 tablespoons water
1 (6-ounce) can apple juice concentrate, thawed
1 teaspoon vanilla
2 cups mixed, chunked fresh fruit

Combine cocoa powder and cornstarch or arrowroot in a small saucepan. Gradually add water to make a smooth paste. Stir in apple juice concentrate. Cook over low heat, stirring constantly until thickened. Stir in vanilla. Place the mixture in a fondue pot or chafing dish to keep warm for dipping. Dip pieces of assorted fresh fruits cut into chunks, such as bananas, apples, pineapple, honeydew melon, or cantaloupe, into the warm sauce.

Hint: Substitute unsweetened orange or pineapple juice concentrate for the apple.

Universal
Conversion
Chart

Measurement Equivalents

Measurements should always be level unless directed otherwise.

⅛ teaspoon = 0.5 mL

¼ teaspoon = 1 mL

½ teaspoon = 2 mL

1 teaspoon = 5 mL

1 tablespoon = 3 teaspoons = ½ fluid ounce = 15 mL

2 tablespoons = ⅛ cup = 1 fluid ounce = 30 mL

4 tablespoons = ¼ cup = 2 fluid ounces = 60 mL

5⅓ tablespoons = ⅓ cup = 3 fluid ounces = 80 mL

8 tablespoons = ½ cup = 4 fluid ounces = 120 mL

10⅔ tablespoons = ⅔ cup = 5 fluid ounces = 160 mL

12 tablespoons = ¾ cup = 6 fluid ounces = 180 mL

16 tablespoons = 1 cup = 8 fluid ounces = 240 mL

Oven Temperature Equivalents

250°F = 120°C   400°F = 200°C

275°F = 135°C   425°F = 220°C

300°F = 150°C   450°F = 230°C

325°F = 160°C   475°F = 240°C

350°F = 180°C   500°F = 260°C

375°F = 190°C

Notes

Chapter 1: There Are Lies and Damned Lies

1. D. Mozaffarian and D. S. Ludwig, "The 2015 US Dietary Guidelines: Lifting the Ban on Total Dietary Fat," *Journal of the American Medical Association* 313/24 (June 23–30, 2015): 2421–22.
2. L. Hayflick, "'Anti-aging' Is an Oxymoron," *Journal of Gerontology A: Biological Sciences and Medical Sciences* 59/6 (June 2004): B573–78.
3. J. McDougall, "Aging in Style: Maybe to 100 with Sensible Care," *McDougall Newsletter,* January 2006, https://www.drmcdougall.com/misc/2006nl/january/060100.htm. G. E. Fraser and D. J. Shavlik, "Ten Years of Life: Is It a Matter of Choice?" Archives of Internal Medicine 161/13 (July 9, 2001): 1645–52.
4. McDougall, "Aging in Style."
5. J. McDougall, "When Friends Ask: Where Do You Get Your Protein?" *McDougall Newsletter,* April 2007, https://www.drmcdougall.com/misc/2007nl/apr/protein.htm; "When Friends Ask: Where Do You Get Your Calcium?" *McDougall Newsletter,* February 2007, https://www.drmcdougall.com/health/education/health-science/hot-topics/nutrition-topics/calcium-dairy-products/.
6. J. Stamler, "The Marked Decline in Coronary Heart Disease Mortality Rates in the United States, 1968–1981; Summary of Findings and Possible Explanations," *Cardiology* 72/1–2 (1985): 11–22; J. Stamler et al., "Dietary Cholesterol, Serum Cholesterol, and Risks of Cardiovascular and Noncardiovascular Diseases," *American Journal of Clinical Nutrition* 67/3 (March 1998): 488–92.
7. J. McDougall, "George McGovern's Legacy: The Dietary Goals for the United States," *McDougall Newsletter,* October 2012, https://www.drmcdougall.com/misc/2012nl/oct/mcgovern.htm.
8. McDougall, "George McGovern's Legacy."
9. McDougall, "George McGovern's Legacy."
10. McDougall, "George McGovern's Legacy."

11. McDougall, "George McGovern's Legacy."
12. Stamler, "The Marked Decline in Coronary Heart Disease Mortality Rates in the United States, 1968–1981; Summary of Findings and Possible Explanations,"
13. McDougall, "George McGovern's Legacy."
14. McDougall, "George McGovern's Legacy."
15. U.S. Department of Health and Human Services, "Overweight and Obesity Statistics," http://www.niddk.nih.gov/health-information/health-statistics /Documents/stat904z.pdf; Centers for Disease Control and Prevention (CDC), "Long-Term Trends in Diabetes," October 2014, http://www.cdc.gov /diabetes/statistics/slides/long_term_trends.pdf.
16. 1U.S. Department of Health and Human Services, "Overweight and Obesity Statistics"; "Obesity Rises Despite All Efforts to Fight It, U.S. Health Officials Say," *New York Times,* http://www.nytimes.com/2015/11/12/health/obesity -rises-despite-all-efforts-to-fight-it-us-health-officials-say.html?_r=0.
17. A. Menke et al., "Prevalence of and Trends in Diabetes among Adults in the United States, 1988–2012," *Journal of the American Medical Association* 314/10 (September 8, 2015): 1021–29.
18. "F as in Fat: How Obesity Threatens America's Future 2012," http://healthy americans.org/assets/files/TFAH2012FasInFat18.pdf.
19. J. McDougall, "The 2015 Dietary Guidelines Are Intended to Confuse the Public and the Press," *McDougall Newsletter,* February 2016, https:// www.drmcdougall.com/misc/2016nl/feb/dietaryguidelines.htm.
20. McDougall, "The 2015 Dietary Guidelines Are Intended to Confuse."
21. J. McDougall, "The Egg Industry: Exposing a Source of Food Poisoning," *McDougall Newsletter,* January 2016, https://www.drmcdougall.com /misc/2016nl/jan/eggindustry.htm.
22. McDougall, "The Egg Industry."
23. McDougall, "The 2015 Dietary Guidelines Are Intended to Confuse"; "The Egg Industry."
24. McDougall, "When Friends Ask: Where Do You Get Your Protein?"
25. J. McDougall, "Protein Overload," *McDougall Newsletter,* January 2004, http://www.nealhendrickson.com/mcdougall/040100puproteinoverload.htm.
26. J. McDougall, "When Friends Ask: Where Do You Get Your Calcium?"
27. J. W. Radshaw et al., "Food Selection by the Domestic Cat, an Obligate Carnivore," *Comparative Biochemistry and Physiology, Part A* 114/3 (July 1996): 205–9.
28. J. McDougall, "Extreme Nutrition: The Diet of Eskimos," *McDougall Newsletter,* April 2015, https://www.drmcdougall.com/misc/2015nl/apr /eskimos.htm.

29. J. McDougall, "Walter Kempner, MD: Founder of the Rice Diet," *McDougall Newsletter,* December 2013, https://www.drmcdougall.com/misc/2013nl/dec/kempner.htm.

30. R. R. Wing, "Cognitive Effects of Ketogenic Weight-Reducing Diets," *International Journal of Obesity and Related Metabolic Disorders* 19/11 (November 1995): 811–16.

31. Q. Zhao, "Detrimental Effects of the Ketogenic Diet on Cognitive Function in Rats," *Pediatric Research* 55/3 (March 2004): 498–506.

32. J. McDougall, "Introduction to New McDougall Book—The Starch Solution," *McDougall Newsletter,* February 2009, https://www.drmcdougall.com/misc/2009nl/feb/starch.htm.

33. McDougall, "When Friends Ask: Where Do You Get Your Protein?"

34. J. McDougall, "People—Not Their Words—Tell the Carbohydrate Story," *McDougall Newsletter,* April 2004, https://www.drmcdougall.com/misc/2004nl/apr/040400pucarb.htm.

35. B. Pobiner, "Evidence for Meat-Eating by Early Humans," *American Scientist,* March–April 2016, http://www.americanscientist.org/issues/pub/2016/3/meat-eating-among-the-earliest-humans.

36. McDougall, "When Friends Ask: Where Do You Get Your Protein?"

37. M. H. Golden, "Protein-Energy Interactions in the Management of Severe Malnutrition," *Clinical Nutrition* 16, Suppl. 1 (March 1997): 19–23.

38. McDougall, "When Friends Ask: Where Do You Get Your Protein?"

39. A. Ströhle, M. Wolters, and A. Hahn, "Carbohydrates and the Diet-Atherosclerosis Connection—More Between Earth and Heaven. Comment on the Article 'The Atherogenic Potential of Dietary Carbohydrate,'" *Preventative Medicine* 44/1 (January 2007): 82–84; author reply, 84–85.

40. McDougall, "Extreme Nutrition."

41. J. McDougall, "A Cesspool of Pollutants: Now Is the Time to Clean Up Your Body," *McDougall Newsletter,* August 2004, https://www.drmcdougall.com/misc/2004nl/040800pucesspool.htm.

42. McDougall, "Aging in Style."

43. R. A. Miller, "Genetic Approaches to the Study of Aging," *Journal of the American Geriatric Society* 53/9 Suppl. (2005 September): S284–86.

44. McDougall, "Aging in Style."

45. B. H. Arjmandi et al., "Soy Protein Has a Greater Effect on Bone in Postmenopausal Women Not on Hormone Replacement Therapy, as Evidenced by Reducing Bone Resorption and Urinary Calcium Excretion," *Journal of Clinical Endocrinology and Metabolism* 88/3 (March 2003): 1048–54.

46. McDougall, "Aging in Style."

47. N. E. Allen et al., "The Associations of Diet with Serum Insulin-Like Growth Factor I and Its Main Binding Proteins in 292 Women Meat-Eaters, Vegetarians, and Vegans," *Cancer Epidemiology, Biomarkers, and Prevention* 11/11 (November 2002): 1441–48.

48. N. E. Allen et al., "Hormones and Diet: Low Insulin-Like Growth Factor-I but Normal Bioavailable Androgens in Vegan Men," *British Journal of Cancer* 83/1 (July 2000): 95–97.

49. Stamler et al., "Dietary Cholesterol, Serum Cholesterol."

50. Stamler et al., "Dietary Cholesterol, Serum Cholesterol."

51. F. M. Sacks et al., "Ingestion of Egg Raises Plasma Low-Density Lipoproteins in Free-Living Subjects," *Lancet* 1/8378 (March 24, 1984): 647–49.

52. McDougall, "The Egg Industry"; "Eggs Are for Easter," *McDougall Newsletter,* March 2005, https://www.drmcdougall.com/misc/2005nl/march/050300 pueastereggs.htm.

53. Stamler et al., "Dietary Cholesterol, Serum Cholesterol."

54. McDougall, "Eggs Are for Easter."

55. J. McDougall et al., "Effects of 7 Days on an Ad Libitum Low-Fat Vegan Diet: The McDougall Program Cohort," *Nutrition Journal* 13 (October 14, 2014): 99, http://nutritionj.biomedcentral.com/articles /10.1186/1475-2891-13-99.

56. J. McDougall, "Results of the Diet and Multiple Sclerosis Study," *McDougall Newsletter,* July 2014, https://www.drmcdougall.com/misc/2014nl/jul /ms.htm.

57. McDougall, "Aging in Style."

58. McDougall, "Aging in Style."

59. D. Buettner, "The Secrets of Living Longer," *National Geographic,* November 2005, http://ngm.nationalgeographic.com/ngm/0511/feature1/.

60. J. McDougall, "Lies and Damned Lies: Damned Lies Harm the Public and Planet Earth," *McDougall Newsletter,* June 2015, https://www.drmcdougall .com/misc/2015nl/jun/lies.htm.

61. McDougall, "Lies and Damned Lies."

62. McDougall, "Lies and Damned Lies."

63. Mozaffarian and Ludwig, "The 2015 US Dietary Guidelines."

Chapter 2: The McDougall Story

1. J. McDougall, "Denis Burkitt, MD, Opened McDougall's Eyes to Diet and Disease," *McDougall Newsletter,* January 2013, https://www.drmcdougall .com/misc/2013nl/jan/burkitt.htm.

2. J. McDougall, "A Brief History of Protein: Passion, Social Bigotry, Rats, and Enlightenment," *McDougall Newsletter,* December 2003, http://www.nealhendrickson.com/mcdougall/031200puprotein.htm.

3. J. McDougall, "The Multiple Sclerosis and Diet Saga," *McDougall Newsletter,* January 2009, https://www.drmcdougall.com/misc /2009nl/jan/ms.htm.

4. J. McDougall, "Walter Kempner, MD: Founder of the Rice Diet," *McDougall Newsletter,* December 2013, https://www.drmcdougall.com/misc/2013nl /dec/131200.htm.

5. J. McDougall, "Nathan Pritikin: McDougall's Most Important Mentor," *McDougall Newsletter,* February 2013, https://www.drmcdougall.com /misc/2013nl/feb/130200.htm.

6. McDougall, "Results of the Diet & Multiple Sclerosis Study."

7. McDougall et al., "Effects of 7 Days on an Ad Libitum Low-Fat Vegan Diet."

Chapter 3: The Healthiest Diet Versus Fad Diets

1. J. McDougall, "The Smoke and Mirrors Behind *Wheat Belly* and *Grain Brain,*" *McDougall Newsletter,* January 2014, https://www.drmcdougall.com /misc/2014nl/jan/140100.htm.

2. T. T. Fung et al., "Low-Carbohydrate Diets and All-Cause and Cause-Specific Mortality: Two Cohort Studies," *Annals of Internal Medicine* 153/5 (September 7, 2010): 289– 98.

3. P. Lagiou et al., "Low-Carbohydrate, High-Protein Diet and Incidence of Cardiovascular Diseases in Swedish Women: Prospective Cohort Study," *BMJ* 344 (June 26, 2012): e4026.

4. H. Noto et al., "Low-Carbohydrate Diets and All-Cause Mortality: A Systematic Review and Meta-Analysis of Observational Studies," *PLoS One* 8/1 (2013): e55030.

5. S. Li et al., "Low-Carbohydrate Diet from Plant or Animal Sources and Mortality Among Myocardial Infarction Survivors," *Journal of the American Heart Association* 3/5 (September 22, 2014): e001169.

6. William Davis, *Wheat Belly: Lose the Wheat, Lose the Weight, and Find Your Path Back to Health* (New York: Rodale, 2011); David Perlmutter, *Grain Brain: The Surprising Truth about Wheat, Carbs, and Sugar—Your Brain's Silent Killers* (New York: Little, Brown, 2013); see also McDougall, "Smoke and Mirrors."

7. J. Montonen et al., "Consumption of Red Meat and Whole-Grain Bread in Relation to Biomarkers of Obesity, Inflammation, Glucose Metabolism,

and Oxidative Stress," *European Journal of Nutrition* 52/1 (February 2013): 337–45.

8. J. Barbaresko et al., "Dietary Pattern Analysis and Biomarkers of Low-Grade Inflammation: A Systematic Literature Review," *Nutrition Review* 71/8 (August 2013): 511– 27.

9. S. H. Ley et al., "Associations between Red Meat Intake and Biomarkers of Inflammation and Glucose Metabolism in Women," *American Journal of Clinical Nutrition* 99/2 (February 2014): 352–60.

10. P. Lopez-Legarrea et al., "The Protein Type within a Hypocaloric Diet Affects Obesity-Related Inflammation: The RESMENA Project," *Nutrition* 30/4 (April 2014): 424–29.

11. S. Hosseinpour-Niazi et al., "Non-Soya Legume-Based Therapeutic Lifestyle Change Diet Reduces Inflammatory Status in Diabetic Patients: A Randomised Cross-Over Clinical Trial," *British Journal of Nutrition* 114/2 (July 2015): 213–19.

12. A. N. Samraj et al., "A Red Meat-Derived Glycan Promotes Inflammation and Cancer Progression," *Proceedings of the National Academy of Sciences USA* 112/2 (January 13, 2015): 542–47.

13. A. J. Gaskins et al., "Whole Grains Are Associated with Serum Concentrations of High Sensitivity C-reactive Protein among Premenopausal Women," *Journal of Nutrition* 140/9 (September 2010): 1669–76.

14. M. Lefevre and S. Jonnalagadda, "Effect of Whole Grains on Markers of Subclinical Inflammation," *Nutrition Review* 70/7 (July 2012): 387–96.

15. D. P. Belobrajdic and A. R. Bird, "The Potential Role of Phytochemicals in Whole-Grain Cereals for the Prevention of Type-2 Diabetes," *Nutrition Journal* 12 (May 16, 2013): 62.

16. Y. M. Lee et al., "Bioactives in Commonly Consumed Cereal Grains: Implications for Oxidative Stress and Inflammation," *Journal of Medicinal Food* 18/11 (November 2015): 1179–86.

17. E. Q. Ye et al., "Greater Whole-Grain Intake Is Associated with Lower Risk of Type 2 Diabetes, Cardiovascular Disease, and Weight Gain," *Journal of Nutrition* 142/7 (July 2012): 1304–13.

18. McDougall, "Smoke and Mirrors."

19. J. McDougall, "Could It Be Celiac Disease?" *McDougall Newsletter,* September 2005, https://www.drmcdougall.com/misc/2005nl/sept/050900celiac.htm.

20. J. McDougall, "Gluten-Free Diets Are Harmful for the General Population (Except for 1 Percent)," *McDougall Newsletter,* March 2013, https://www.drmcdougall.com/misc/2013nl/mar/gluten.htm.

21. T. A. Kabbani et al., "Body Mass Index and the Risk of Obesity in Coeliac Disease Treated with the Gluten-Free Diet," *Alimentary Pharmacology and Therapeutics* 35/6 (March 2012): 723–29.

22. W. Marcason, "Is There Evidence to Support the Claim that a Gluten-Free Diet Should Be Used for Weight Loss?" *Journal of the American Dietetic Association* 111/11 (November 2011): 1786.

23. McDougall, "Gluten-Free Diets Are Harmful."

24. McDougall, "Smoke and Mirrors."

25. J. Cheng, P. S. Brar, A. R. Lee, and P. H. Green, "Body Mass Index in Celiac Disease: Beneficial Effect of a Gluten-Free Diet," *Journal of Clinical Gastroenterology*, April 2010, 44(4):267–71. doi: 10.1097/MCG.0b013e 3181b7ed58.

26. McDougall, "Smoke and Mirrors."

27. J. McDougall, "Simple Care for Diabetes," *McDougall Newsletter,* December 2009, https://www.drmcdougall.com/misc/2009nl/dec/diabetes.htm.

28. J. McDougall, "Walter Kempner, MD: Founder of the Rice Diet," *McDougall Newsletter,* December 2013, https://www.drmcdougall.com/misc/2013nl /dec/131200.htm.

29. H. A. Wolpert et al., "Dietary Fat Acutely Increases Glucose Concentrations and Insulin Requirements in Patients with Type 1 Diabetes: Implications for Carbohydrate-Based Bolus Dose Calculation and Intensive Diabetes Management," *Diabetes Care* 36/4 (April 2013): 810–16.

30. McDougall, "Smoke and Mirrors."

31. A. G. Henry et al., "The Diet of Australopithecus Sediba," *Nature* 487/7405 (July 5, 2012): 90–93.

32. J. Mercader, "Mozambican Grass Seed Consumption during the Middle Stone Age," *Science* 326/5960 (December 18, 2009): 1680–83.

33. A. G. Henry, A. S. Brooks, and D. R. Piperno, "Microfossils in Calculus Demonstrate Consumption of Plants and Cooked Foods in Neanderthal Diets (Shanidar III, Iraq; Spy I and II, Belgium)," *Proceedings of the National Academy Sciences USA* 108/2 (January 11, 2011): 486–91.

34. A. Revedin et al., "Thirty Thousand-Year-Old Evidence of Plant Food Processing," *Proceedings of the National Academy Sciences USA* 107/44 (November 2, 2010): 18815–19.

35. L. Liu et al., "Paleolithic Human Exploitation of Plant Foods during the Last Glacial Maximum in North China," *Proceedings of the National Academy Sciences USA* 110/14 (April 2, 2013): 5380–85.

36. M. Mariotti Lippi et al., "Multistep Food Plant Processing at Grotta Paglicci (Southern Italy) Around 32,600 cal B.P.," *Proceedings of the National Academy Sciences USA* 112/39 (September 29, 2015): 12075–80.

37. J. McDougall, "The Paleo Diet Is Uncivilized (and Unhealthy and Untrue),"
     McDougall Newsletter, June 2012, https://www.drmcdougall.com/misc
     /2012nl/jun/paleo2.htm.

38. Loren Cordain, *The Paleo Diet: Lose the Weight and Get Healthy Eating
     the Foods You Were Designed to Eat,* rev. ed. (Hoboken, NJ: Wiley, 2011);
     McDougall, "The Paleo Diet Is Uncivilized."

39. K. Milton, "Hunter-Gatherer Diets: A Different Perspective," *American
     Journal of Clinical Nutrition* 71/3 (March 2000): 665–67.

40. Personal communication by Nathaniel Dominy, Ph.D., recorded at the
     McDougall Advanced Study weekend, September 9 to 11, 2011, Flamingo
     Resort, Santa Rosa, California.

41. McDougall, "The Paleo Diet Is Uncivilized."

42. K. Hardy et al., "The Importance of Dietary Carbohydrate in Human
     Evolution," *Quarterly Review of Biology* 90/3 (September 2015): 251–68.

43. McDougall, "The Paleo Diet Is Uncivilized."

44. E. Carbonell et al., "Cultural Cannibalism as a Paleoeconomic System in the
     European Lower Pleistocene," *Current Anthropology* 51/4 (2010): 539–49.

45. J. McDougall, "Extreme Nutrition: The Diet of Eskimos," *McDougall
     Newsletter,* April 2015, https://www.drmcdougall.com/misc/2015nl/apr
     /eskimos.htm; "Calcifications of Mummies' Arteries Due to Meat in Their
     Diet," *McDougall Newsletter,* April 2013, https://www.drmcdougall.com
     /misc/2013nl/apr/fav5.htm.

46. McDougall, "Extreme Nutrition."

47. A. Ströhle, M. Wolters, and A. Hahn, "Carbohydrates and the Diet-
     Atherosclerosis Connection—More Between Earth and Heaven. Comment on
     the article 'The Atherogenic Potential of Dietary Carbohydrate,'" *Preventative
     Medicine* 44/1 (January 2007): 82–84; author reply, 84–85.

48. J. McDougall, "An Inconvenient Truth: We Are Eating Our Planet to Death,"
     McDougall Newsletter, December 2016, https://www.drmcdougall.com
     /misc/2006nl/dec/truth.htm; "Human Health and Planet Health—Same
     Solution," *McDougall Newsletter,* January 2007, https://www.drmcdougall
     .com/misc/2007nl/jan
     /warming2.htm.

49. R. Goodland and J. Anhang, "Livestock and Climate Change," *World Watch
     Magazine* 22/6 (November/December 2009): 10–19.

50. M. Springmann et al., "Analysis and Valuation of the Health and Climate
     Change Cobenefits of Dietary Change," *Proceedings of the National Academy
     of Sciences USA* 113/15 (March 21, 2016): 4146–51.

51. McDougall, "The Paleo Diet Is Uncivilized."

52. McDougall, "Th e Paleo Diet Is Uncivilized."

Acknowledgments

There are a number of individuals who were instrumental in making this book happen. I am grateful to all of the following for sharing in my vision and bringing this book to life: Cathy Fisher, Carole Bidnick, Gideon Weil, Miles Doyle, Hilary Lawson, Sydney Rogers, Melinda Mullin, Laina Adler, Terri Leonard, and the team at Girl Friday Productions.

Index

Note: Italic page numbers refer to illustrations.

and *McGovern Report*, 6, 7
risk of, 4, 15, 38, 51, 76, 116, 122
treatment of, 39
and vegetable oils, 122–123
carbohydrates. *See also* low-
carbohydrate diets
complex carbohydrates, 7, 16, 18
false association with type 2 diabetes,
63–64
and human nutritional needs, 14,
15, 18
importance in human evolution,
69–70
simple carbohydrates, 16
sources of, 16, 17, 18, 55, 60
carnivores, *88*
carrot soups. *See also* soups
as green-light food, *105*
celiac disease, 57–63
Chana Masala, 199–200
cheese, as red-light food, *99*, 122
Cheezy Baked Macaroni, *183*,
201–202
Chinese people, 18, 27, 38–39
Chittenden, Russell Henry, 42
Chocolate Fruit Fondue, *198*, 251
cholesterol
in animal-based foods, 2, 11, 12, 13,
19–23, 88, 120, 121, 122
cholesterol levels, 21–23, 26–27, 29–30,
31, 37, 46, 96
chronic diseases linked to, 5, 11
and Healthiest Diet on the Planet,
30, 31
and *McGovern Report*, 7
and Paleo Diet, 71
sources of, 13, 22–23, *22*, 26
USDA guidelines on, 2, 10–12,
21–22, 33

chronic diseases
cholesterol intake linked to, 5, 11
and Healthiest Diet on the Planet,
16, 32
history of, 27
and *McGovern Report*, 7
risk of, 4–5, 38
and starches, 64
treatment of, 39, 41–42
cold cereal, as green-light food, *102*
constipation, "food poisoning" as cause
of, *85*
conversion chart, 253–254
Cordain, Loren, 67–68, 70, 72–73
corn
Creamy Corn Soup, 143
as green-light food, *110*
corn syrup, 17
Costa Rican Potatoes and Beans,
203–204
couscous, Israeli Couscous Salad,
171–172
cranberries, Pear-Cranberry Crumble,
196–197, 247–248
Creamy Corn Soup, 143
Creamy Golden Gravy, 235
Crunchy Quinoa Salad, 167–168, *186*
Curried Yam Stew, *187*, 205

dairy foods. *See also* animal-based foods
macronutrients in dairy compared
to meat, *123*
Davis, William, 53, 60–61
degenerative diseases, 4–5
Department of Health and Human
Services (DHHS), 2–3, 10, 11–12
desserts
Banana-Strawberry Delight, 250
Berry Sorbet, *195*, 246

Permissions and Credits

Recipe photographs by Jennifer Davick Photography

Screen capture of Dr. McDougall's article (page 95): © McDougall et al.; licensee BioMed Central Ltd. 2014. This is an Open Access article distributed under the terms of the Creative Commons Attribution License, which permits unrestricted use, distribution, and reproduction in any medium. http://nutritionj.biomedcentral.com /articles/10.1186/1475-2891-13-99

Other photos by:

p. 79: © Natykach Nataliia/Shutterstock; © Gregory Gerber/Shutterstock; © Nattika/ Shutterstock; © Jiang Hongyan/Shutterstock; © MaraZe/Shutterstock; © Stockvision/ Shutterstock; © szefei/Shutterstock; © Yeko Photo Studio/Shutterstock; © Oliver Hoffmann/Shutterstock; © Igor Dutina/Shutterstock. p. 82: © Luis Louro/Shutterstock; © Dml5050/Dreamstime. p. 83: © pixelheadphoto/Shutterstock; © Chaowalit/ Shutterstock. p. 84: © Peter Kotof/Shutterstock; © Andrea Danti/Shutterstock. p. 85: © Denys Prokofyev/Dreamstime. p. 86: © 914 collection/Alamy. p. 87: © DVARG/ Shutterstock. p. 88: stockphoto mania/Shutterstock; © Oleksandr Homon/Dreamstime. p. 89: © sevenke/Shutterstock. p. 90: © Private collection/Bridgeman Images. p. 91: © casejustin/Shutterstock. p. 92: © Luis Louro/Shutterstock. p. 93: © Robyn Mackenzie/Shutterstock; © stockcreations/Shutterstock. p. 94: © Nikolay Petkov/ Shutterstock. p. 95: © McDougall et al. licensee BioMed Central Ltd. 2014. This is an Open Access article distributed under the terms of the Creative Commons Attribution License, which permits unrestricted use, distribution, and reproduction in any medium. http://nutritionj.biomedcentral.com/articles/10.1186/1475-2891-13-99. p. 96: © Gregory Gerber/Shutterstock. p. 97: © Jiang Hongyan/Shutterstock; © Cloud7Days/ Shutterstock. p. 98: © Carlos Romero/Shutterstock; © Nattika/Shutterstock. p. 99: © Luisa Leal Photography/Shutterstock; © azure1/Shutterstock. p. 100: © ziviani/ Shutterstock; © aspen rock/Shutterstock. p. 101: © Valentyn Volkov/Shutterstock. p. 102: © Telecast/Dreamstime; © Pamela D/ Maxwell/Shutterstock. p. 103: © MaraZe/Shutterstock; © Jennifer Davick Photography. p. 104: © Bhofack/Dreamstime;

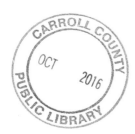